W9-DDN-599

I AM NOT MY BREAST CANCER

WILLIAM MORROW *An Imprint of* HarperCollins*Publishers*

I AM

not

MY BREAST CANCER

Women Talk Openly About Love & Sex,
Hair Loss & Weight Gain,
Mothers & Daughters,
and Being a Woman with Breast Cancer

Ruth Peltason

FOREWORD BY Peter I. Pressman, M.D., F.A.S.C.

I Am Not My Breast Cancer is based on an online dialogue created by Marc N. Weiss and Ruth Peltason and hosted by Web Lab.

This book contains advice and information relating to health care. It is not intended to replace medical advice and should be used to supplement rather than replace regular care by your doctor. It is recommended that you seek your physician's advice before embarking on any medical program or treatment. All efforts have been made to assure the accuracy of the information contained in this book as of the date of publication. The publisher and the author disclaim liability for any medical outcomes that may occur as a result of applying the methods suggested in this book.

HarperCollins books may be purchased for educational, business, or sales promotional use. For information please write: Special Markets Department, HarperCollins Publishers, 10 East 53rd Street, New York, NY 10022.

FIRST EDITION   362,196 99449

Designed by Janet M. Evans

Library of Congress Cataloging-in-Publication Data has been applied for.

ISBN 978-0-06-117410-0

08   09   10   11   12   WBC/RRD   10   9   8   7   6   5   4   3   2   1

For my grandparents,
Ruth M. and Paul E. Peltason

I see dark nights and beautiful sunny days.
I see the seasons changing with a feeling of hope.
I am a hawk, soaring over the world and brushing
those I love with the wind from my wings.
I see myself committed to making the world a
better place, striving to help those in need
of healing and succor. I see hurt and anger
sometimes, but mostly cheer and good humor.
I see life. I see myself, forever and always.

> —*Gwendolen R. Leighty ("songbird"),*
> 1955–2005

Contents

Foreword

I Am Not My Breast Cancer is a book that will help women realize that they are not alone when dealing with this disease. It will help their families, friends, colleagues, and also their physicians—anyone who is part of the fabric of their lives. It is a book that addresses what women are really feeling during this time when their health is at risk and their emotions are running high. It touches on the feelings they have about themselves head-on, with no compromises and no punches pulled.

I suspect that anyone who reads this book will be somewhere along the road of discovery, treatment, or recovery from breast cancer. It addresses the reactions a woman with breast cancer will have at these different stages as well as the responses of those around her. It is not designed as a repository of medical facts. I have written books for women about breast cancer and believe these professional guides are important. But even the most responsive and compassionate physician—male or female—cannot provide the enormous range of personal support women can provide to one another.

If you are lucky enough to have a friend who has been through treatment at your side, that can be a terrific asset. That's rare, however. Some women find it useful to attend support groups. But for others, the spectrum of personalities among women and the unpredictability of the weekly agenda may be daunting and not helpful. The session you attend may be focused on the subtleties of breast reconstruction when you may be concerned about imminent hair loss or how to tell your teenage daughter what's happened. How do you find the group that is right for you?

The Internet is another source of information, and the stories of other women's lives can be at your fingertips. But this takes time at the keyboard and a lot of searching—no matter how computer savvy you are, you might end up in the wrong chat room or not be able to find what you need. This book recognizes the value of the Internet as a resource and is based on the author's Web project named *First Person Plural*. Ruth Peltason, who has had breast cancer, has read the stories of hundreds of women who took part in that project. Her achievement in *I Am Not My Breast Cancer* is to have woven these voices into a compelling narrative that speaks boldly to what women feel during this time. Her book is organized so that you can easily read the contents and focus on the experiences other women have had in very specific areas that may be your current concern.

No one person can tell you how to react, behave, and manage personal or medical encounters. Everyone has a specific style. We read novels because authors have the ability to enlighten us with insights into other peoples' lives. Here, Ruth Peltason provides an ongoing, cohesive narrative, making it much more than a collection of questions and answers. The book is a sharing of emotions combined with a lot of medical facts, too. There is the reality of the side effects of medical treatment, as well as how the diagnosis and treatment of cancer are handled differently by family, friends, and coworkers—and also how others may react to you. You can read it from cover to cover, or you can concentrate on the topics that are most beneficial to you. In either case, the book will be there for you according to your needs.

Some people say the experience of having cancer transformed them; it certainly does change your life, at least for a while. During that time, it is useful to have a book close by that, while it will not have your name in the index, has a table of contents that reflects your journey. It is also comforting to take solace from and to learn from the experiences of others.

Peter I. Pressman, M.D. F.A.C.S.

Introduction

B y the time I was in the fourth grade, I had a stack of dreams: I wanted to be a teacher, baton twirler, model, writer, artist, and have a springer spaniel farm. None of these dreams included being someone with breast cancer.

Fast forward to when I was thirty-five, going for my first mammogram. To be honest, I didn't even know what getting a mammogram actually involved, so when I was told to raise my arm, lean forward, and not breathe while my breast was sandwiched between a cold, viselike thing (what I now call the "mammogrammer"), I thought it was pretty weird and barbaric. It was also painful. And when I was told that more images were needed, it didn't occur to me that this was unusual; I didn't even bother to ask why. Looking back, the period between those last images and when the radiologist, Julie Mitnick, walked in and spoke to me marked the shift from innocence to loss. In real time it was only a few minutes, but for me it was an eternal gauntlet thrown down: You have cancer. You might die. Today your life will change.

Breast cancer is one of the most democratic diseases. Regardless of a woman's education or bank account, where she lives, whether she's pretty or nice or highly moral, today one in eight women is diagnosed with breast cancer; 85 percent of them have no family history of the disease. Indeed, in women the only cause of death greater than breast cancer is lung cancer. When I consider my breast cancer alongside these facts, I'm just a blip on the screen, a number among other numbers. When I was thirty-five, I recall, one in nine women would get breast cancer. At the time I had about eight to ten close girlfriends, so I figured that if I was taking a bullet for the group, it wasn't so bad. My lumpectomy sure wasn't a mastectomy, and having radiation was in no way like chemo, so it was a piece of cake, a *morceau de gâteau* that I could handle. I was never mad, I never felt that God was punishing me or that bad karma or kryptonite was raining down on me. I was not, I told myself, Chicken Little or Pigpen, and I was not going to say the glass was half-empty when it still looked half-full.

Over the next dozen years I had additional biopsies, not pleasant, but not overly worrisome, either. But then my luck changed, or the cancer recurred, or *something*, because in my late forties Julie Mitnick again said, "I have some bad news for you." And this time I was out of wiggle room: a mastectomy, reconstruction, and chemotherapy followed. So did hair loss, dry skin, and aching joints. And a tremendous sense of loss and worry. I was also bewildered. When my brother Jim asked if I felt like "why me," I replied, "No, but I wonder, 'Who—*me?*'" Surely they had the wrong girl. I was the little drum majorette, the high school track star, the overachiever, the girl who got the boys. Wrong. Now I was the girl who got breast cancer, and I didn't like it one single bit. I didn't feel like I'd survived anything, I just felt shitty and alone.

That's when the idea for this book kicked in. I'd been home from the hospital for a few days and my sister-in-law, Barb, was staying with me to help out. It was about two a.m., she was asleep in the next room, and I was trying to get out of bed. *Trying* because part of my abdominal muscles had been cut during the tram flap procedure, so I didn't have the strength to go from a prone position to one sitting up, and so I was stuck, with my legs hanging off the side of the bed. I was just sort of rocking, like a turtle on its back, and in pain. "This is ridiculous," I thought, "I can't even get out of bed by myself." Yet instead of having my own little pity party in the dark, I realized that if I was having a hard time, even with a great support system of family and friends, and some of the country's best doctors, what about women whose lives were harder? What about women who had children to get dressed and off to school in the morning? Or what about women who lived miles away from their doctors and a good hospital? Or women whose husbands or partners weren't supportive? Or had employers who weren't sympathetic? Worse still, what about women who were flat-out alone? I knew I wanted to do something, and I resolved to write a book that would speak to all of us. I would write the book I couldn't find, for women I didn't know but who, like me, were struggling with life issues.

I'm a nut for books, and one overall addiction I claim is an appetite for too many interests, hence too many books. Yet, weirdly, I only owned two books about breast cancer, both of them medical guides—one by my surgeon, Peter I. Pressman, and one by Dr. Susan Love. To me, the other breast cancer books seemed too saccharine or superficial, a little too "la-di-da," as Annie Hall would say. I wanted the warts-and-all, tell-all sort of book that focused on how women with breast cancer dealt with undressing—with a lover or in a locker room at the gym; what it was like losing your hair (and not just on your head) and having it come back in; whether women gave up careers or pursued them harder; whether humor helps and worrying about mortality hinders. Was there any proverbial silver lining in the breast cancer cloud or was it just rain, rain, rain? Was anyone else afraid to buy green bananas?

While I was going through chemo, friends often came by to help out or to provide good cheer. One evening Marc Weiss, the husband of one of my best friends, came by. (Marc's wife, Nancy Meyer, and I grew up in St. Louis, and in New York we live only a few blocks from each other.) I was telling Marc that there was no book that really spoke to me about the so-called big issues of living with breast cancer—and certainly not to the degree that I craved. Marc has a well-regarded Web company that produces online dialogues about important social issues, and after a little brainstorming we hatched a plan to work together and combine our skills. From the start, it would be a two-part project: Marc and I would develop a website, and I in turn would adapt it for the book that I felt was needed. We decided that only women with breast cancer could participate—no siblings or parents; no husbands, partners, or friends; no doctors or therapists. Simply stated, this was a "members only" club. The Web project, named *First Person Plural* and formed with the help of ten leading breast cancer organizations, advisers, and funds from many generous souls, was launched two years later. Wobbly, perhaps. Idealistic— most certainly.

After we hosted the Web project I began reading the comments, sorting through the material, and making the selections for this book. What you are holding is easily one-fifth of the rich bounty I had to consider. Ultimately, I must have read thousands of stories told by eight hundred women. This extraordinary number of women—by far the largest to date in any book on the subject of living with breast cancer—comes from every state in the country, as well as from Canada, Europe, Australia, and Africa. Racially, they are white, African-American, Hispanic, African, and Asian. They range in age from their early 20s to their late 70s. Some of them are dealing with pre-cancers, whereas others are dealing with metastases or are terminally ill and coping with all that entails. Yet they all benefit from connecting with women who have breast cancer. Although their communications were frank and intimate, they used pen names ("screen" names in computer lingo) to preserve their real identities. They signed their notes with these names and used them when addressing one another. After a while, writing to "Blue Girl" seemed as natural as using "Anne" or "Lucy," and so this form of identification is carried forward in this book. Significantly, I think this privacy permitted the women to reveal some of their deepest feelings (the warts-and-all element), especially when talking about their families or sexuality or, say, aspects of their childhood. What you read here are the original texts, with a little spit-polish—in editing the women's comments, I did my best to preserve individual cadence and voice, limiting myself to corrections of spelling and grammar, typos, and tightening of passages for impact and considerations of length.

For the most part, I felt that the comments succeeded without further annotation (and distraction) from me to the reader, although the chapters "Children" and "When You Look in the Mirror, What Do You See?" are exceptions to the rule. Here I added brief biographical information because I felt that age or family history, to cite two such examples, was especially relevant to some of the entries.

I Am Not My Breast Cancer is authored by ordinary women with breast cancer for readers everywhere who are dealing with breast cancer and its many personal and symbolic ramifications. The women included here work in factories, are stay-at-home moms, secretaries and CEOs, teachers and nurses. They are blue collar and white collar; atheists and believers; straight and gay; single, married, divorced, and widowed. Some work two or three jobs; others are newly retired. Women who have traveled the world swap stories with those who have never left the small towns where they were born and raised. Language and writing skills vary. I applaud the similarities and the differences, for these are the real voices of women everywhere doing their honest best to communicate, share, and learn. They support one another, they grieve together, and they have what they call "group hugs." (One woman, who lives in a remote community in the northwest, wrote that for the first time she didn't feel alone. It was also the first time in ten years that she'd ever talked about having breast cancer.) I am immensely proud to introduce readers to my eight hundred new friends. Sadly, in the course of assembling this book, some of the women who participated in the online project and whose comments are here have since died. They are cherished and deeply missed.

As everyone who's been diagnosed with this disease knows, sometimes the only constant or enduring help is from other women like us. Nothing is more isolating than finding out that you have breast cancer, and the sympathy we get from friends or family only goes so far—typically it's intermittent and often freighted with other issues.

Even the status of loved ones as "outsiders" never changes. Women with breast cancer thrive on connecting with other women who speak the same language and share the same concerns. The help and nurturing they offer one another is its own reward.

I Am Not My Breast Cancer has been organized in three parts, which loosely chronicle the progression of living with breast cancer. Part 1, "Diagnosis," begins with receiving and sharing the news of a diagnosis, and includes the many feelings one experiences (anger, depression, stress, coping, et cetera), hair loss, and being at work. Part 2, "Living with Breast Cancer," focuses on primary relationships for women: with their spouses and lovers; as mothers and daughters; and with family, friends, coworkers, in-laws, even pets—which one woman aptly called her "fur babies." The material here about sexual intimacy is remarkable for its candor and depth: no one pussyfoots around delicate topics, although more than one woman remarked she was glad the comments were anonymous (ditto for her husband!). If you've ever wondered how someone else felt when making love following a mastectomy, or how other women dealt with a spouse who seemed to shut down, or about other young women struggling to have children after chemotherapy, you will find it here. The last section of the book, "The Big Picture," addresses the significance of anniversaries and milestones; the role of religion and spirituality; and mortality. For me, the chapter "When You Look in the Mirror, What Do You See?" is the most moving: more than two thirds of the women responded to this call for a frank assessment of themselves. Their written self-portraits are full of heart and honesty. Imagine the courage it takes for a woman diagnosed at the age of thirty-four and put into chemical menopause to write, "When I look in the mirror I see a future." And imagine the humanity expressed here: "When I look in the mirror I see every other woman who has gone through this."

The overall optimism expressed by the women in these pages is one of the unexpected revelations I had while working on this project. Woman whose lives were hard as dirt distinguished themselves with dignity and grace; women who'd had to terminate a pregnancy managed to smile through their tears; and women who had previously lost a sister or a mother or an aunt to breast cancer remained defiantly positive. I'm no scientist, but I'm tempted to say that women naturally have an inner buoyancy and resiliency.

On a more political front, these voices are a wake-up call: we need to overhaul the mind-numbing and dehumanizing health insurance for women in this country. Not one woman in this book was satisfied with her health insurance—and that's a shameful statistic. Having a diagnosis of breast cancer is hard enough; actually having to persuade some anonymous health insurance clerk to approve what the companies have decided are out-of-network services—mammotome biopsies, surgery for tram flaps, nipple reconstruction, or breast symmetry, for example—is humiliating. And exhausting. Should a woman really have to fight for a surgery that allows her the dignity of having her post-operative breasts look the same size? Should a woman have to forfeit some household item so she can pay for much-needed care by a psychotherapist to alleviate anxiety or depression? For some women, this struggle becomes the factor that finally breaks their spirit. This is wrong. I believe we can and should do better.

My greatest wish for this book is that it offer comfort to any woman living with breast cancer and to those who care about her. If this book is kept on the bedside table, then I hope its need is brief and its impact lasting. *I Am Not My Breast Cancer* speaks of courage, heroism in deeds small and large, and incredible faith and fortitude. Even the title of this book underscores an unwillingness to be defined by disease. As Alexander Pope, the great eighteenth-century English poet, wrote, "Hope springs eternal in the human breast." How true, and how nobly this is displayed in the hundreds of comments included here, for in books no voice is ever hushed and dreams never end.

Ruth Peltason
New York, New York

PART ONE

Diagnosis

CHAPTER ONE

Sharing the News

"How do you tell your family news you can
barely comprehend yourself?"

lovinglife

There was nothing laudable about how I learned that I had breast cancer: the surgeon who performed the biopsy literally said, "I'm so surprised. You have a malignancy," as I was walking into his office and before I'd even closed the door. Welcome to my world. I had just turned thirty-five. (Ironically, I had been humming an old Streisand tune "Happy Days Are Here Again" on my way to the doctor's office—indeed!) In the couple of seconds it took this doctor to speak, my life was forever changed. That was also the last time I ever heard an ill-spoken word from a doctor and marked the first time I took my care into my own hands—I changed surgeons and have been happy ever since. But back to that day: after the appointment I went to my office and called one of my best friends. Without skipping a beat, she came immediately—we cried, and then I left the office without saying a word and took off the rest of the afternoon. I remember we went out for lunch.

To this day, however, I still can't recall the specifics of calling my parents in St. Louis to tell them I had breast cancer. For one thing, I *remembered that my mother's brother died at the age of fifty-four from bone cancer and that my grandparents felt a lifelong sadness because of that. Was I going to die before my parents, too? Weren't children supposed to outlive their parents? My father's response was simple and direct: "Come home" and be treated there; I was already very uncomfortable having the discussion, but I stood my ground, saying that I felt the best doctors were in New York. What else? I'm sure they asked questions; I'm sure I tried to answer those I could.*

Jump ahead twelve years. I had a recurrence and this time the stakes were higher. And by this time my father had passed away. Again, I called that same best friend. Maybe she called my mother; maybe I called my brothers. Maybe some variation on this occurred. It was not a happy time, and I was weirdly calm, in that calm-before-the-storm sort of way. As for my friends and colleagues: I think the news trickled out, on a need-to-know basis. Memory, as I have learned, can be an unreliable witness.

Sharing this kind of news is an active process fraught with emotion. As a sign of modern technology, often the most efficient (and least stressful) way to communicate is by e-mail, typically with the so-called calmest family member designated as "sender." Understandably, the following accounts detail highly charged experiences. And while the conditions are similar—the women have just learned they have breast cancer—their stories are unique.

FAMILY

I just wished my mom wasn't by herself when she was told. She lost her husband of 48 years to cancer and then me getting it was like a nightmare. I can only imagine what she is feeling, but I know how horrible it would feel if one of my children were diagnosed with any kind of cancer. My youngest daughter came to see me later that evening and as soon as I saw her I started to cry and told her I have never even flown a kite so I was going to fight this with all I could. She as-

sumed the role of mother and was there during my emotional out-
bursts and helped me to gain my composure.

lilybelle2

My mother-in-law cried every time I talked to her. That was very upsetting for me. I felt I had to comfort her instead of the other way around.

ritavv

I had to tell my parents over the phone as they were on vacation and
that was so hard. It makes you cry twice, because you have to all cry
again when you see each other.

Michele

My husband was a seven-hour drive away on maneuvers with his Air
National Guard unit. I got him on his cell phone and told him that I
might have cancer and to stand pat. I might need to have the Red
Cross bring him home. (My wonderful husband was by my side a day
later.) My parents were local. They were out of the house and on the
way to the doctor's office within 5 minutes and we all waited for me to
go in to have the ultrasound.

I so didn't want to scare them, but I was scared and needed my
mommy and daddy there. When the results of the ultrasound showed
positive for cancer, we had a group hug and they held me as I cried.
Then I held my mom as she cried—her mom had died of breast cancer and she always taught me to be vigilant in preventive measures.
My eyes met my dad's and I became resolute that I would beat this.
He'd been through too many tragedies in his life—he lost his whole
family in the gas chambers of Treblinka. I would *not* have him lose a
child. That was simply not an option.

CarynRose

Since my sister had died from breast cancer in 1986 at age 43, my
husband had been secretly waiting for "the other shoe to drop." My

husband, who is very protective of me and has been my soul mate for the last 33 years, assumed the job of the "teller." He broke the news to our sons, which was so difficult for him. My close girlfriends, who are like family to me, took the news so very hard. They were with me through my sister's horrific illness and they saw what it did to me. They were not sure I was strong enough mentally to make it through the same horrendous treatment again. But, I guess I found out that I'm stronger than anybody thought I was. Now, 5½ years later, my doctors tell me that I am well and healthy. I am truly a lucky girl.

> Swanky Sue

When I called my sister, who isn't the brightest tool in the shed, God bless her, she asked me immediately, "Are you going to die?"

> Marybe

When I was diagnosed after my biopsy I didn't want to tell my family until after I had my next surgery so I would have a better idea of what to tell them. The night after I got home my sister called me and said "Oh, I just had to call you. I had the strangest dream, I dreamed I was fighting with our brother Sean because he said he was going to take you away from us!" You see, my brother died of AIDS in 1993. Well, at that point I told her and we cried together. I then decided to tell my other brother who was working on a cruise ship in Alaska. When I called him he said, "I had a weird feeling something was wrong. I was standing on the dock and something on a park bench kept flashing in my eyes; when I looked to see what it was, it was the same saying that we had put on our brother's headstone painted in gold." I believe that my brother Sean was helping me to contact everybody. When he was alive he would nag me about calling everyone to stay in touch. The saying was from an *Alice in Wonderland* poem that he liked: "Lingering in the golden gleam/Life, what is it but a dream?"

> B-Positive

I have 2 sisters, 9½ and 11½ years older than I. Our mother was diagnosed with breast cancer in 1977, my oldest sister in 1997, and I in 2000. My oldest sister was away from home that weekend, and my mom "unreachable" because of her Alzheimer's. After telling my brother/boss, I called my other sister to tell her my news. She didn't say anything for a while, then very quietly said, "It's supposed to be *my* turn." I had to cry, because she was an X-ray tech who had had 8 surgeries on her back and neck. I told her that if I got a vote, she'd miss her turn on the breast cancer; so far, she has!

    HopeNFaith

The hardest ones for me to tell were my father and my children, ages 14 and 11 at the time. I wanted to be able to give my kids some concrete information, not just "Mommy has cancer but we don't know anything else." Especially since they lost their grandmother to breast cancer, I knew this would be scary for them and I wanted to right away be able to give them some facts as to how my case was different. While I never have brushed off the cancer to the kids, I also have been very open and casual about it.

    buckeyemom

I was very worried about telling my father of my cancer diagnosis because my 63-year-old mother had just died after a 2-year battle with lung cancer 6 weeks prior to my diagnosis. Actually, truth be told, I felt the lump in my breast while in the shower on Mother's Day 1991 when I was taking care of my dying mother at her home. I kept the news of my breast lump to myself because of everything that was happening. The only person I shared this news (and my worry) with was the hospice nurse who was helping us care for my mom. I had an excisional biopsy with frozen section that revealed my cancer diagnosis on the spot. I was so prepared for this diagnosis because my mother had breast cancer at 35 and I had just celebrated my 34th birthday the week before. Since my mom had just died, I really needed to tell my father in person. I arrived at his home with my brother unannounced and he was startled. I knew he knew something was very wrong. We sat down and I told him the good news was that I felt well, and the not-so-good news was that I was just diagnosed with breast cancer. Here's the most amazing response I got spontaneously from him: "Well, Dolly, if you have at least 26 years like your mother had after her breast cancer then you will be ahead of the game." I was surprised that he could pull out this response. Having just lost his wife of 43 years I expected a different response.

Eileen

Some families start out in denial . . . and remain that way

I didn't call my family until I returned home from the hospital. As predicted, they were in denial about the whole thing and still pretend it didn't happen.

Doreen

> "My mother has taken it well, but she is one to deny things."
>
> SacredHeart

I called my sister. I am very, very close to her. While we were talking, her husband was online reading, researching, and telling me good sites that he found about my type of cancer. My sister remained one of the most important parts of my support team. Then I called my mother who is a 12-year survivor of the same type of breast cancer that I had (DCIS). Her response was sooooo strange. I was crushed. She asked almost no questions. She didn't offer to come help, nothing. I think that because of her history maybe it was just too hard for her to deal with right off.

Mom continues to be a mystery. She will answer my questions but won't elaborate, won't tell me how she felt or any of that. When I complained early on about being lopsided she sent me a catalogue about prostheses and bras, but that is about all.

Nett

HUSBANDS AND SIGNIFICANT OTHERS

When I was diagnosed, my partner of 10 months was in the room with me. His former wife died from uterine cancer so I thought surely he would want out of our relationship. Instead he sent flowers to my office with a card saying he was in this for the long haul however long that may be. We were married a year later. A new chapter started for me when I met my second husband. Since I was diagnosed around the same time, one positive effect has been to highlight how grateful we feel that we met.

kyra

The news was hardest on my husband. I think for the first time in our thirty-plus years of marriage he couldn't fix it or make it go away. I had to go through this and there wasn't anything he could do to change that.

Gram K

> "Telling those that love me that I had cancer was by far the most dreaded thing I had to do. Not the half a dozen surgeries, not the chemo, not the radiation."
>
> MoxieAir

My husband is a loner, a Silent Sam, who said little. But he's steady as a rock and has continued to treat me the same as always. I never ask him to look at my body, but I do undress in the same manner as always, and he touched my incision site once, in the dark, ever so gently. I asked him once what he thought of men who would leave a woman at a time like this and his answer was, "I'm not that shallow." End of discussion.

Mawsquaw

Guess who also needs support? Your spouse

"Still waters run deep" would be another way of describing what happens to men when their mate is diagnosed—they may seem *quiet, they may* seem *like they're holding everyone together, but in fact* they *need some attention, too. It's important to remember that what happens to you also happens to your husband.*

After everything was done and over and the focus was off *me*, I finally had time to really take a good look at my husband and was sorry to see that he had very little support through all of this. Everyone was always hovering over me and busy giving me support that now I feel bad that he really did not voice his concerns or have his own support network. At the time, I was actually mad at my husband because he seemed to withdraw from me and as things got tougher, he was less and less supportive. He worked longer and longer hours and was gone many weekends, hunting and coaching. After a while, he did not even know what was going on with me. He stopped asking and a wall went up between us. A year after the largest part of my ordeal is over, I am just starting to understand how awful he felt—he had to "go into his cave" and get away from the pain of it all. My sister-in-law was the only one who understood this as she was with him when he received my grave diagnosis after many hours in the waiting room. He held up until the children left and then he collapsed into her arms and just sobbed and sobbed. My husband never cries and is not one to discuss his fears. I wish that we could have shared our fears together. I am happy to say, though, that after I had a meltdown, things have improved significantly and we are communicating much better. It really took things to get to a crisis point for me to start talking like we should have all along.

newday

I was furious with my husband in the beginning. How could he not understand? He didn't appear sympathetic enough for me. Of course, he was working 12-hour shifts during my chemo treatments and was exhausted when he came home. He worked 7AM to 7PM and took the best care of me that he could. I didn't stop to think of the pressure it put on him until he broke down and cried and told me he felt helpless. I knew then that I couldn't depend on him completely and had to get involved with a support group. People who understood what I was going through took pressure off of him because I wasn't looking to him for all my support. He's a loving father, a hard worker, and we're getting along just fine now.

1Faith

My significant other struggled with his desire to be there for me and my desire to remain independent. When things settled down, we talked and he told me that he felt that I had really shut him out. I was so focused on being strong and minimizing the effect cancer had on my life, that I really didn't tune in to the fact that allowing him to be a little more involved might have helped him cope.

uneven but breathin

My husband went with me to every chemo treatment, but he spent most of the time pacing.

jillbers

My husband was really good throughout just about everything. The occasional time when I'd mention fear of dying or anything about dying at all (which was very rare, really) he'd accuse me of being negative. I realized those fears were just something he was not comfortable discussing. He didn't care if I lost my breast, lost my hair, or whatever, as long as I was still alive. Death was just one aspect he could not face.

bradleyteach

CHILDREN, WITH A SPECIAL FOCUS ON TELLING YOUR DAUGHTERS

Telling your child you have cancer goes against every natural instinct that a parent has, especially with young children. Instead of protecting you are now causing them to worry; instead of nurturing you are causing hurt; instead of preserving innocence you are hastening feelings of loss. In a matter of minutes, your children go from seeing you as invincible to seeing you as very, very mortal. All of this is compounded for women with daughters. Sadly, these discussions take place in homes across America every day.

> "While I have never brushed off the cancer to the kids, I have also been very open and casual about it."
>
> buckeyemom

We told our kids, 9 and 4 at the time, that mommy has cancer and that in killing the cancer it would kill other things in my body like my hair. This scared them a bit. We told them that the hair would come back, but the cancer would not. I would not do anything differently. And I think we did the best that we could have with the children, given their ages.

junebugs

My kids did not know about all the activities pre-diagnosis. We waited to tell them since my son had a starring role in his middle school play that week and my daughter was taking SATs on that Saturday. After her SATs we all had lunch together and broke the news then. They were upset—my daughter quietly so (we have a classic mom-daughter tense teen relationship) and my son visibly upset. I was able to reassure them by pointing out kids they know whose mothers have been through what I was going through. Still it was difficult. I think it was almost harder to tell my mother who, since she was widowed a few years ago (my father died of lung cancer), has become pretty dependent on me. I told my kids that it was fine to share this news with anyone they wanted to. This helped them. My daughter received a tremendous amount of support from school friends and got to know kids who said "oh yeah my mother went through that when I was in such and such grade." I also relied on the grapevine, and the outpouring of support was really touching. I've always thought being open with these things brings more benefits than negatives. My experience with breast cancer has proven this to me once again.

    stellaluna

The hardest thing I had to do was talk to my kids, 2 daughters and a son, all in their 30s and long since left home. I thought about not telling them until I had something certain to tell them but decided that if they knew the possibility of cancer, it would be easier to accept the reality. You've got to know that I'm an old Italian mother who can't move past the mothering part to friendship with my adult children. I probably drive them crazy with help and suggestions—correct that: I do drive them crazy. My son (the youngest) was very analytical, wanting to know chapter and verse. The girls were stunned at first but very positive. I decided not to tell anyone else until I had a few more facts.

    januss

My husband was with me for the news, and we told various friends and relatives. The one that stands out for both of us was our daughter, our only child, 10 at the time, and the center of our lives. We told her all we knew, answered her questions, and let her teacher know to keep an eye on her. She and my husband started doing "Daddy-Daughter Days" on the day after chemo, to leave me home to rest. (She's 19 and they still have an occasional Daddy-Daughter Day!) She was 15 when it recurred and we told her whatever she wanted to know and kept her updated. I worry that she is too concerned about me, and if I don't report what the docs say or test results are, she calls me from school to ask. But there is a good side to this: she is compassionate to others and she doesn't treat ill people as if they are diminished for their illness or disability.

Toni

The hardest talk was with my two grown daughters. I told the doctor that I didn't know how to tell my daughters and how I felt I'd dealt them a rotten card. He just looked me in the eye and said, "You can tell your daughters that you did nothing wrong, you've taken care of yourself and that there is no place for blame or guilt. You're going to get through this and while their fears are real and they should talk about them, do not accept any *blame* for what has happened." I'm usually pretty straightforward and not afraid to stand alone if I have to, but this experience rattled my confidence quite a bit.

MT

Telling my girls was the hardest thing I have ever done. Both handled it well, but my youngest daughter gave me the best compliment I have ever received. She told me, "Mom, this is the first time I ever realized that you are mortal, and I want you to live until my children are grown." Interestingly enough, she didn't have any children at the time of my diagnosis, and it took three tries and two miscarriages before she had her first beautiful little boy.

Mawsquaw

I called my daughters the day after the diagnosis, but (typical of me) I assured them that it was contained in the breast and I would be fine.

My older daughter knew better and helped me out by doing a lot of research online to help me decide between a lumpectomy and a mastectomy. My younger daughter was more naive (and I didn't provide much information, mea culpa) and almost passed out when she saw me in my room after the surgery. I will be much more forthcoming if I have a medical problem in the future.

lindaslegacy

BEING ALONE

The day after I had my mammogram and biopsy, I got the phone call from my gynecologist, whom the surgeon had called with the results. When she said "your test came back and it was cancer," I remember I was sitting on the bed all alone and I felt like I was going to be sick, and for a few hours I kept drifting in and out, wondering did I just hear what I thought I heard. I waited awhile and then I called my twin sister who lives in another state. She made me promise that I would call my cousin (who lives nearby) so that she would be there with me since I'm not married. She has been there with me from the very beginning, going to every chemo treatment and doctor appointment.

river

> "I wouldn't change the way I handled anything, except believing I was invincible in the first place."
>
> Sara C

Two days after Christmas I received a phone call while I was at work from my surgeon. It was around lunchtime. I remember screaming and was comforted by a nice lady who worked in my office. It was only us in the room. I didn't automatically call anyone to tell them. I had to leave work immediately.

I don't remember driving home. It was the most surreal experience I could ever have imagined. I was truly on autopilot. I still get chills when I think back to that horrific day. If there are any doctors reading this, *please* do not call your patients at work to tell them the news. I could have gotten into a car accident on the way home and couldn't have waited long enough to have anyone pick me up. I needed to be home.

To this day I regret the fact that my surgeon, who I respect dearly, broke the news to me over the phone at work. I wish she would have called me at home, or had asked me to come in. I was in complete and utter shock that it was cancerous. I was only 32.

reginabu

After finding a lump, having a mammogram, ultrasound, and a biopsy, the nurse at my doctor's office called to schedule an appointment the next day, telling me not to worry. I never dreamed I'd hear the word *cancer* so I went to this appointment alone. Only my husband and a couple people at our business knew I was having tests.

I was numb. Totally stunned and could hardly speak. My doctor offered to call my husband for me as I didn't think I could actually get the words to come out. He had a coworker bring him to the doctor's office and we just truly held each other for a long time knowing our lives were about to change.

I went to see my parents to deliver the news. I felt I needed time alone with them. It was a difficult discussion and I could tell how scared they were. I involved them all the way. My mother once again took me under her wing and was always there when I needed her to be. She is always so giving and positive. I felt 10 again instead of 41.

I wouldn't change the way I handled anything, except believing I was invincible in the first place.

Sara C

A COMPANY OF ONE: KEEPING THE NEWS TO YOURSELF

Does this hearken back to being "a good girl" and not bothering anyone? I think so. It certainly resonates for me.

> "Not sharing the illness with those close to you doesn't allow them to deal with it and get the pleasure of helping you."
>
> JoAnn

I didn't want to be the newest soap opera episode at work or church, so I kept my issue under the roof of my house. People are so self-absorbed that very few noticed a change in me. For the few that did suspect, I simply said I was fighting off something and was a bit tired. I'd end with, "You know how it is," and invariably they'd say yes and proceed to tell how they too seemed to be fighting off some kind of virus. (I didn't lie to anyone. Believe me, I really was fighting.)

Delivered

There are a lot of people in my life whom I have not told about my breast cancer. Unless they ask in a sincere way how I am I just don't bother to share.

pat

> "I didn't want to be the newest soap opera episode at work or church, so I kept my issue under the roof of my house."
>
> Delivered

I told as few people as I possibly could. I didn't tell my father until after I was done with chemo. I never told cousins, aunts, uncles, next-door neighbors, my babysitter/housekeeper who had worked for me for several years at that point, the teachers at my child's nursery school, the mothers of her friends, or most of my friends. I only told three people at the job that I'd worked at for twenty years and I told them they couldn't discuss it with anyone else. I told my husband he could tell one or two people at work; I told my mother-in-law she couldn't tell any of her friends that knew me save one, whose daughter was a cancer survivor. I have never disclosed or discussed being a cancer survivor with any of the above people or with anyone else in my community, other parents at my child's school, or anyone in my church. Is that strange or what?

For almost a year I couldn't talk about breast cancer without crying, so that was a major reason. And I also felt right from the beginning that the only people who could possibly understand and therefore the only people worth talking to were fellow survivors. Five years later, while it has been weighing on me recently having this big secret, I'm not sure it was such a bad approach. The few times I've told people, I've regretted it. People are mostly either scared or morbidly curious and they are in complete ignorance or denial about the reality of breast cancer. I was too and never knew what to say to people before I was diagnosed. The few people in my life who know don't want to talk about it. I'm very happy not to be the breast cancer poster girl in my office or professional life, community, social circle, church, etc. Of course, if I heard about anyone in my life who was diagnosed with breast cancer, I would talk to her immediately and share my experience or help her in any other way I could.

Annie

I never share my breast cancer experience with anyone. No one close to me really wants to know much about it. It seems like the minute I had my last chemo it was *done*, I was supposed to be fine. Well, the longer I try to assume that disposition the harder I struggle with all of the info we are all exchanging. I am usually feeling very misunderstood by my family and friends. Just how does a person try and relate all the physical and emotional behavioral patterns we seem to all suffer? I am not a person who whines; I was just raised to be tough and get going. Somehow that theory is not working for me now. My family really loves and cares for me, but they are not available for this part. My sister was a blessing also but she's moved on from this too. Seems like I am not supposed to say anything at all, just that I am fine. That's pretty far from the truth as far as the drama I am finally feeling. My self-image is a mess.

Bren

FEELINGS OF REGRET

I put off telling my family who live in another state, two brothers and an aunt, my mother's younger sister, because I didn't know how to say it. Well ironies of ironies, I got a call from my cousin one day who said she had some bad news to tell me. I replied to her I too had some bad news to report. She told me my oldest brother had died of a blood clot to his heart. This almost broke me. I told her my news and then said I have to go now. I needed to release my grief: I cried and cried and cried. My older brother would always call and check on us and he was the only one, now he was gone and I didn't call him because I didn't want to tell him about me. I regret putting that call off so much. It was dumb to put it off, so I would advise all to tell those you are close to so you can all help support one another.

NMRose

I had no problem telling anyone but my mom. She was going through chemo for her lung cancer and my family said I should not tell her about my cancer. My mom was my best friend throughout all of my life—we had a relationship that was the greatest gift God ever could have given. She knew something was wrong because I wasn't going over to see her. I waited almost two weeks, and then asked my cousin to please tell her for me. It should have been me who told her, and I should have told her when I first found out. My family was selfish for asking me not to and I should not have listened to them. I was my mother's rock and she was mine. We gave each other strength.

　　Autumn

Make a decision and don't look back and regret what you have done. You did the best that you could do at that particular moment.

　　Linda

DON'T BE AFRAID: SHARE THE NEWS

> "I decided that the more people that knew the more prayers I would get."
>
> 　　lilybelle2

I found it very, very difficult to share my news with any of my family. Being a very independent person I thought that this was my cross to bear and to not complain. After all, there were always people worse off than me. Because I was to be at a family celebration the day I had my biopsy, I had to mention why I would not be there to my family. Of course once it was out everyone knew!!! But you know what? It was the best thing that could have happened! And I say to anyone who thinks that she can manage on her own, give your families and friends a chance to show their love and support! They want to be included in the bad news as well as the good news. I bore the bad news for three weeks and I know looking back that I would not have done as well with the "whole world" on my shoulders.

　　Nemo

"No, I am not blessed to have this d#$@ disease, but I am truly blessed to be surrounded by so many people who love me and care and want to see me through."

Scottie

I am a professor at a small school and had just been elected president of the faculty senate. I called thirty people in a classroom and told them myself. Thirteen seconds later it was all over campus. I am glad I went public. I was not ashamed, I had done nothing wrong and quite frankly, I could use all the good thoughts any one of them could send my way. People were afraid for me, but it helped me be less afraid for myself.

playwright

BEING UPBEAT

"Whenever people asked me if I was okay, I would tell them no, but I will be."

river

A friend of mine who was with me when I found out it was cancer told everyone if they couldn't put a smile on their faces don't go see me. And you know, they were great—all I saw were smiles and I believe that helped.

faith

It was difficult to tell my parents. My mother had always been so emotionally fragile, that I wanted to present the news in an upbeat manner. When I told them, I was very positive and did not express any concern. I believe that presenting the news in that manner was beneficial to my mother and assisted in keeping her from falling apart.

clk913

> "I had no trouble talking about it as long as I didn't have to actually say 'I have breast cancer.' That would make me cry every time."
>
> PattiT

It's funny how you can be so terrified and feel so vulnerable, and yet feel that you have to be the strong one in the family for everyone else.

PugAddict

From the start I was in a daze but also was being strong for everyone else. That is what I did through the whole thing it seems—be strong for everyone else. Any other emotions of fear or pain I kept to myself most of the time. The hardest was telling my best friend of 29 years. She has had breast cancer, in remission 12 years, but she has lost most of her family because of it. She took it hard, and now with my recurrence she has taken it even harder. She tries to hide how she feels, but I know. I know.

SacredHeart

THE BENEFITS OF BEING OPEN

One of the unexpected "joys" of being upfront about a diagnosis is that sometimes you meet other women who've experienced the same thing. Suddenly you go from being a group of one to being part of a group of many . . . and what a comfort that can be!

"As the saying goes, 'To know the road ahead, ask those coming back.'"

Kim W

One of my best friends has had the dubious honor of going ahead of me in the breast cancer battle, and her example of openness made it easier for me to decide how I want to include others in my own journey.

Lizzi

I did not have any trouble telling anyone about my diagnosis. I think being open makes others more comfortable around you, and makes them aware of their own health. A lot of women I work with scheduled mammograms after they heard about me. A very interesting thing happened to me after my diagnosis. My friend's mother had a 70th birthday party. She invited some old college buddies from Long Island. I was sitting at a table full of breast cancer survivors! I asked them many questions—nothing was too personal. This was the best thing that could have happened to me. One woman even showed me her scar. Because of this, I wasn't afraid when my bandages came off.

Peony

After my diagnosis 4 years ago I have always felt the responsibility of helping others going through their cancer and sharing my cancer experience with others. I remember how terrified I was when I was diagnosed and how much it meant to me when women who I hardly knew came up to me and told me that they had survived. As the saying goes, "To know the road ahead, ask those coming back." I feel that we are the ones coming back and I feel we can help those women starting that long road.

Kim W

PASSING THE NEWS ALONG: PLAYING TELEPHONE

After a while, I just couldn't tell any more people because I hated making them feel so sad and scared for me. Yet I wanted friends to know. My solution was to write a poem. I picked out pretty paper to print it on and added a little personal note as well. It seemed like a gentler way to break the news.

Traveling Girl

> "There is no good way to tell someone they have cancer!"
>
> pinkwings

I am the baby of six kids and my father died of cancer when I was very young. I knew my mother would have a very hard time so I used a phone tree method (all my family live about a 17-hour drive away). So I phoned the person who I thought would be the most practical and be able to keep their cool—my sister-in law. I told her the situation and I asked her to ensure that she told my mother in person.

My mom called. It was terrible but we got through it. Then they started a phone tree to tell the rest of my family and friends that lived close to them. Then we had to start the calls to all the friends. You know, by then I was very practical, to the point and very factual. I think I went into automatic. People were shocked, crying, etc., and I was consoling them. Go figure. I just got so used to saying the same thing over and over that it wasn't registering anymore. I think I also ran out of tears by the tenth call.

Fun Lover

I did use e-mail to formally tell my family and friends after the news was out. To be honest, I know that I talked to my brothers and my husband's brothers too, along with my grandmother and aunts, but I honestly can't remember a lot about it. I continued to keep family and friends informed via group e-mails, and that helped a lot with not having people call all the time, or having to send a bazillion individual e-mails.

buckeyemom

If things keep happening to you over the years, you have to make judgment calls on whom to notify when, or whether to notify some people at all. For instance, my husband, family, and closest friends hear most everything, but a bit further outside the circle, I don't usually report test results (unless dramatic) or other things unless I happen to be talking to the person. You can really get yourself jammed on the information highway if you try to communicate to too many people, but I think you can get yourself seriously jammed emotionally if you don't tell enough people (# to be decided by oneself, of course).

Daisy

CANCER ISN'T A DEATH SENTENCE: THE PITY LOOK

Some people would look at me like I was already given a death sentence and I could see the pity in their eyes so I avoided people like that. One of my coworkers told me she felt sorry for me and I got mad and told her I didn't want her pity, I wanted her prayers!!!! My sister-in-law, the one I'm closest to, would not even come to see me—she avoided family functions and everything if she knew I was there. She told me later if she didn't see me then she wouldn't have to think of the cancer. So you just never know how some people will react and certainly not the way you would expect them to.

lilybelle2

I found that I couldn't be the one to tell people. I had my husband do it for me. I guess I was afraid of seeing the "she's going to die look" in their eyes. Most people are not knowledgeable about breast cancer and assume you're going to die if you get it. I just didn't need that.

ritavv

SURVIVORS: A HELPING HAND

Outside of my dear husband and daughter, my support came from an unexpected source: my Internet friends. I've been corresponding with a large group of sewing buddies since bulletin boards first came about. I've had the opportunity to meet many of these women when we attend sewing conferences around the country. These are women from all walks of life and all ages—some work full time and some are stay-at-home moms. Many are grandmothers and some are never married or newly single. I decided to let my Internet friends know so I started a discussion thread titled "I have breast cancer." I explained what was happening and my dear husband posted on the day of my surgery to let them know how it was going. The support I received from these women is unbelievable. One of my Internet friends organized a "shower of cards" as a total surprise to me. The week after my surgery when I went to get the mail, the mailbox was full of cards and letters and little gifts from my Internet buddies! And what's more, it continued for nearly a year! I didn't find out until about a month ago that she just asked everyone to send a card or note once a month on the date of their own birthday so it was easy to remember.

In this day and age of e-mail and telephones, we don't remember the thrill of getting letters and believe me, it was wonderful beyond belief. It has made me very good about remembering to send a card or jot a note when I'm thinking of someone.

Little Dutch Girl

I am a very verbal person. I don't think there is anyone out there that knows me, or knows about me, who doesn't know I had breast cancer. One of the positives is that people (both men and women) come up to me for information (either for themselves or for someone they know). It is a way to open doors and let people know that you can survive cancer and live a wonderful life. I am a 14-year survivor.

I am also very active in 2 support groups, one of which I co-facilitate. I was so glad to have a place to go and talk about what was happening to me and my body that I want to be able to give others that same safe haven.

I know that chat rooms and message boards are the "thing" to-day. I do check them out occasionally to see what's new. But for me, there is nothing like the hugging, holding, touching, laughing, crying, etc., found in a live person-to-person group. I will be involved for as long as I am able.

smilie

CHAPTER TWO

Crowning Glory: Hair Today, Gone Tomorrow

> "I suppose losing my hair made me come to terms with myself more."
>
> Nushka

W hen I was a teenager, my girlfriends used to say that my hair was like a lion's mane—thick and wild. It more or less remained that way until I began treatments for chemo. I remember being incredulous when my oncologist told me that my hair would fall out—how could that happen to me, the girl with all the hair? In preparation for that fateful time, a friend and I went wig shopping and found ourselves at what I came to affectionately call "the wiggeria." It was just off the Garment District and mainly provided wigs for Orthodox Jewish women. The woman who helped me was kindness itself. She was also unequivocally confident: "You will be beautiful, my dear. Of this I am sure." I went all-out and got a terrific head of someone else's hair, and took it to my own stylist to have her cut and shape it.

Once my hair started to go (it happened while I was in my accountant's office—I ran my hand through my hair and was aghast to realize that the hair on my head was now clumped in my hand), I decided to be proactive and take some measure of control over its demise. I called a friend, who came over with her husband's clippers and shaved my head. To my surprise, it felt pretty great. I wore my wig for months and took loving care of it, just as I had fussed over my dolls' hair when I was a girl and played "beauty parlor." Whether I looked beautiful, as promised by the Wig Lady, is debatable; what I can say with her unequivocal confidence is that I never had a bad hair day. But I definitely did not like windy days.

Women who undergo chemo are nearly unanimous in their unhappiness about losing their hair. As one woman writes, "When my hair started to come out I freaked. It was the first real image of cancer to me." By extension, for some women, losing their hair is a double whammy: first their breast, then their hair. What next? For others, being bald is a badge of courage and they sport their new hairless do's with confidence, even exuberance. There is even something humorous about losing your hair—sort of. More intimate still is losing hair elsewhere on your body—not just your eyebrows and eyelashes, but down there. *Now that is unsettling!*

RITE OF PASSAGE—BOTH GOOD AND BAD

It was springtime and when I finally called a friend to come over and shave my head, it seems my need for cleanliness outweighed my need for privacy. I told her I wanted to shave my head in the backyard so we wouldn't have to deal with the mess. I figured it would go fast and we'd be back in the house in a flash. We took a kitchen chair outside and my friend started shaving my head. Well . . . my backyard isn't that private and my friend's husband and 8-year-old daughter were out walking their dog when they saw us and decided to come over. (They didn't realize what was going on. They were just being their normal, friendly selves.) Then my boyfriend came home early with my son and they came out looking for me. (I never told them that I wanted privacy.) Then my next-door neighbor, who was out walking his 2 dogs came over to find out why all the people were milling around in my backyard. It never occurred to any of them that this might be awkward for me. They were all just so fascinated to see a woman having her head shaved in the backyard that they were treating me like some kind of star performance artist.

As I sat there on that kitchen chair that spring evening, half-bald, looking up at my friends and family who were surrounding me, I didn't know whether to laugh or cry. Finally I decided to laugh. It was just too absurd. As I think back I realize that sometimes when the little things don't go the way you plan, ya just gotta roll with it.

Tracy43

> "If one more person tells me 'it's just hair,' I'm going to whip scissors out of my backpack and tell them I think *they'd* look great with short hair, too."
>
> Agent99

Before I started chemo, my oncologist told me that 2 weeks after the first treatment, I'd start losing my hair. Well, exactly two weeks to the day, after that first round, my best friend and I were driving home from running errands. It was a beautiful day out, mid-70s, blue skies. We were driving with the windows down, when I noticed my hair slipping out of my head and out the window! I screamed, "Shelly, my hair is falling out," as I was shutting the window. But Shelly opened the window to watch my hair fly out. We were both pressing the window control button, me to close it and she to open it. All the while we were laughing hysterically.

My hair, which is extremely thick, was coming out in handfuls, usually in the shower. After about a week of letting it come out on its own, another friend (she's my hairdresser and her mother had recently died of lung cancer) shaved my head.

I didn't wear a wig. I had a couple of lovies-style hats (a local church group makes and donates them to breast cancer patients) and some scarves that I wore. Even though I was cerebrally prepared for my hair falling out, and had gone through that with my stepfather, my father-in-law (both had lung cancer) and my dad (who had brain cancer), there was still that initial shock, the disbelief. It was very visceral, standing in the shower with clumps of hair in my hand.

Once I was bald, I really enjoyed it. I just loved rubbing my head while I read. It was so calming, it felt sensuous (in a non-sexual way). My husband would yell at me to "stop obsessing with my head." For Halloween, I dressed up as Uncle Fester from the *Addams Family*, light bulb and all.

KeyWoman

My hair was down to the middle of my back, curly and full. My *best* feature!!!! As I knew that it would fall out, I cut it short after the surgery and when it started to fall out, 2 weeks after the 1st treatment, I went to the hairdresser who has been doing my hair for nearly 15 years. After the store closed, she shaved my head. It was almost like a ritual. We both cried but knew that it was a temporary thing. I bought a very expensive wig and rarely wore it. It was too uncomfortable. I wore hats and one day decided to go to school "in the raw." My students thought that it was the coolest thing and asked me not to wear hats anymore.

My hair has grown in thin, straight, and sparse. I went from not being able to see my scalp to very thin hair. But I am alive and healthy and that is a very small price to pay. I also lost my eyelashes and eyebrows and they have also grown in thin and sparse. The hair in my legs came back with a vengeance!!! Isn't it ironic??

graciela0107

I was so worried about losing my hair. I'm one of those people if my hair didn't look good I felt like s—t. So this was a big thing for me. My hair was poker straight to my shoulders. I loved wearing my ponytail. I had my hair cut short and everyone said you look so cute. I told them well then I'll be even cuter when I'm bald! Cancer gives you lots of joke material. I went and got the most expensive wig possible and wore it once. I felt so unlike me. Luckily it was summer and we spent a lot of time at the pool, so I wore bandanas. Once summer was over I was so tired of putting things on my head that for the rest of the time I just walked around bald. It actually made me feel better.

The worst was when I started to lose my eyebrows and eyelashes. That's when I started to look like a cancer patient.

beth

Oddly, losing my hair was not that big of a deal for me. While I had the normal angst about how hot and uncomfortable the wig was and hard to find the right style, I actually liked not having to shave my legs and losing the other unwanted body hair. So many women shave or shape their pubic hair that this didn't bother me either. I went wigless at home and am fortunate to have a nice head and looked good in extremely short hair. I will certainly miss the extra time I had every day in not styling it as well. Knowing it was temporary I decided to enjoy the upside.

ScaredSilly

When my hair first started growing in and was super-short, like a buzz cut, people would walk up to me on the street every day and compliment me. I think other women assume you have a certain independent personality to have that haircut or something. Anyway, that was okay, but I *hate, hate, hate* my hair at this stage of growing out. It's short and curly and I feel like I have an old lady haircut. If one more person tells me "it's just hair," I'm going to whip scissors out of my backpack and tell them I think *they'd* look great with short hair, too.

Agent99

When I started to lose my hair with chemo, I called my hair guy and asked him to shave my head. We had a blast, pics and everything, cutting my hair first into a mohawk, then into little knobs. At the end, we hugged and he cried. When I got home, my partner said, "You look like G.I. Jane (Demi Moore's character in the movie)." That said, I put on a gray T-shirt and shorts and prompted myself into what "appears" to be a three point/one-arm push-up, similar to G.I. Jane. We took pics and gave them to family and friends. I felt really great taking control over the hair loss/chemo.

mac

THE PUBLIC YOU

> "You think that everybody is going to be looking at you, but they don't."
>
> googie

I wore a wig only if going out someplace special, otherwise the turbans and other little hats were great, as was just going out without anything! You'd be surprised how many people really don't care, not even looking twice. You think that everybody is going to be looking at you, but they don't. My hair was straight as a board, but now it came in curly and I love it and keep it very short! It's a lot softer too, but still a lot of it/thick.

googie

I don't know about you, but dealing with the baldness has been very difficult. In the beginning, I wore a wig and was always worried about how people would react to my baldness. Of course, as the hot flashes began, more and more, the wig came off; I found I didn't care any longer what people thought.

One friend saw me at a banquet: I had my wig on, got hot, and took it off. The next day at work she said, "I saw this beautiful bald woman at the banquet last night and thought 'that lady has cancer, I should pray for her.'" Then she said that she kept thinking the lady looked familiar. "Then I realized it was you and that I do pray for you!"

    ally

My absolute worst has happened twice now. I had my 3 small children in a restroom while traveling home for Christmas. I was so anemic and neutropenic and just felt like crap. Not one hair to be found anywhere on my whole body. This *rude* woman, as I was walking out of the restroom after fighting my kids to not touch *anything*, says, "Sir, this is a ladies' room." My mouth flew open in shock, but my darling 5-year-old says loudly, "Mommy, that lady's stupid. She doesn't know about cancer hair." She was mortified and I was so glad. The other one was a pizza-faced kid at McDonald's who called me "sir." I was wearing a pink scarf, pink sweater, and makeup that time.

    kimmytoo

I was out one night with *very* short hair; it had just started growing back. A guy was walking by (complete stranger) and asked "Oh, why did you chop all your hair off?" All I said was "cancer, a**hole" and kept walking!

    lou_nc

I had just found the courage to take my wig off and start wearing my new short hairdo to work. A lady (who obviously did not know my story) announced, "Girl, why in the world did you cut your hair?" I politely told her that I had been wearing a wig and went on in detail about having breast cancer. Her response: "Well, you should put the wig back on. It makes you look younger."

    LaurieV

DOUBLE WHAMMY: FIRST THE CANCER, THEN THE HAIR LOSS

Losing my hair was the defining moment that it was *true*. I really had cancer and was really taking chemotherapy. It was very traumatic and devastating for me. My hair had been one of my best features. My doctors had told me it would come out approximately two weeks after chemo started, but I thought I would be one of the lucky ones and it would not come out. I was wrong. I refused to shave my head and allowed each strand to fall out.

Blessed

> "When my hair started to come out I freaked. It was the first real image of cancer to me."
>
> MJ

I hated losing my hair and had it cut real short before it fell out. I bought two wigs and looked pretty good. The wig lady was fabulous—she reminded me that most people are so wrapped up in themselves that they don't notice other people anyway. I went to my son's wedding 8 months after chemo sans wig (it was hot and my hair was short but it looked okay). My hair came back great. It is curly and very thick. I actually like it better, though I could have done without the whole experience.

Traveler

It's great that some of you can speak so positively about losing your hair. For me, it was nearly as traumatic as receiving the breast cancer diagnosis. While I was prepared for losing it about two weeks into chemo, the actual experience was very difficult for me. When my hair started coming out, I called my mother and just cried.

Ellen

BALD IS BEAUTIFUL: A BADGE OF COURAGE

> "Being bald has helped people come up to me and talk."
>
> memphisgirl

Losing my hair was definitely a difficult time. Prior to that time I had cancer but I didn't have the *look*. Some long pieces remained and I eventually shaved all the leftovers off. I did get a wig before my hair came out but I never felt it was me and I only wore it once for a few hours and stuck with bandanas and baseball-type caps and a knit cap on those cold winter nights. I did have a picture taken of myself with my bald head and wearing a T-shirt that said "I'm too sexy for my hair that's why it's not there," and did send it to friends and family that have been supporting me through all of this ordeal. It helped me to be able to say, "Hey, I'm okay even though I have no hair."

fuzz top

Baldness was not a big deal for me, however I started chemo beginning of winter so was real bald when it was terribly cold. Outdoors I wore a beanie and took it off when I was indoors. It didn't raise any eyebrows with most people as they knew my family is originally from Lesotho. People in Lesotho, as part of their culture, keep bald heads. I have photos of when I was bald. I take them out to remind myself of this unique journey.

Kgadi

I think a woman who is bald from chemotherapy (or anyone for that matter) is wearing a *trophy* of her triumph. It's temporary, and a sign that better things are happening.

rooter

"Hey, I'm okay even though I have no hair."

fuzz top

My husband helped me a lot, dealing with my hair loss. He would kiss my head and rub it saying he loved my bald head. That would make me laugh.

Jean

Being bald has helped people come up to me and talk. I guess they think, "She is bald, she must be okay talking about it." I cannot believe the people who needed someone to talk to, so I consider this to be a reason for having cancer twice. I am an experienced listener and advice resource. I have met so many wonderful people that I never would have even noticed or they would have never noticed me had I not been bald.

memphisgirl

HAIR TODAY, GONE TOMORROW

My hair was longer than shoulder length when I started chemo. I was optimistic for a few weeks since no loss was apparent, but I brushed my hair out of my face one day, and that was it—it all came out. I just kept running my hand through my hair, and within half an hour, all of my hair was no longer attached to me! Strangely, I stuffed it all into one of those grocery store plastic bags. And I still have it, eight years later. Don't know why, but I just can't part with the hair!

Stillhere

I didn't save all my hair, but I did save a long lock of it. Now my hairdresser has it and uses it to try to color my hair back to what it was like before. Some people are so happy to do whatever they can. The woman who does my hair would not accept any payment the day she shaved it off, nor did she charge me when I went it to get the "shaggies" trimmed when it started to grow back. In fact, I didn't cry when she cut off all my hair, but I did when she said she wasn't going to charge me for it. The woman at the shop where I got my wig didn't charge anything for the fitting or the wig styling and only charged me her cost for the wig itself. She made absolutely no money off of those transactions and basically donated her time. These are just 2 examples of people who wanted to help and found a meaningful way to do so.

kamaha

"The answer, my friend, is blowin' in the wind . . ."

When I started my chemo I went and bought a short wig (my hair was a little longer than shoulder length). A few days later, I took scissors and cut my hair in layers to almost resemble the wig. I wanted a smooth transition for my family and myself. When my hair did start to fall out I let the wind grab it for the birds also (there must be some soft and colorful nests up in the trees).

tuppie

I love the idea of letting the birds use it for their nests. When mine started to really fall out, I woke up one morning and sat there pulling it out in clumps, making a pile on my lap. My husband was getting ready for work and would pass me by and give me strange looks. I wouldn't look into a mirror until I was done. Then he started smirking. When I looked in the mirror we had a good laugh. I have kept my hair in a baggy to compare it to what grows in now. Just for fun. When I'm done I think I will go in my backyard and let it blow in the wind for the birds.

Beth's still smiling

NO MORE BAD HAIR DAYS

Call it vanity, call it a crutch, call it an attempt to hold on to your dignity—wearing a wig to cover being bald is great, with two exceptions: going swimming and being caught in a wind tunnel.

I had a beautiful wig and I used to joke about what it must feel like to be a Vegas showgirl, putting on my face, my brows and liner . . . and when the wig was on I felt complete again. Showtime! That was my coping mechanism. Wearing it made me feel as though I wasn't sick because many people couldn't tell, and I didn't want stares and pity . . . and yes, okay, I was vain! I had a boyfriend when I was diagnosed, but the relationship didn't make it, and I was in great turmoil over my appearance during that time.

Eventually, I actually had a problem parting with my wig, because my hair was long and blond and so was the wig. The wig actually looked better than my real hair! When it grew back in short, black, and curly, I couldn't bring myself to take off the wig because then I realized everyone who hadn't known would suddenly be on to me. What a pickle! I even had 2 longtime friends gang up on me in a restaurant and drive me to tears because they told me I needed to deal with who I really was and stop hiding. (Needless to say, my social worker told me to rethink those friendships.) I think I have learned quite a lot about myself and others from all this.

Nushka

I am one of those people more comfortable with a wig. I had one to start with and now I have a total of five. I could cover my head and look normal but you can't disguise missing eyelashes and thinning eyebrows and that really bothered me. I did learn the trick to use eyeliner on the upper and lower eyelids which helped a lot, and my coworkers really never realized I lost my eyelashes.

Polish Princess

HAIR COLOR

RedBird, kamaha, and Nushka talk about the change in color when their hair grows back.

How do others feel about the change in hair color when it comes back in? My hair was always dark brown with red highlights, now it is black with white highlights. My wig is dark brown with red highlights, so most people don't know I've been through cancer treatment and hair loss. They certainly will know when I quit wearing the wig and show up with short, straight, black and white hair. Is this just a vanity issue, a 'I can prove I can get through this' issue or an 'I have a right to keep my health issues to myself' issue? I'm okay with my new color at home and with close friends but just can't seem to get over the hurdle of taking the wig off for work, church, etc. Having spent 7 months with the wig I may have become attached to my crutch, but summer is here and it is too hot to wear. Has anyone colored/dyed her hair when it was new? Does it work?

RedBird

RedBird,

My case was different because I almost always wore a baseball cap or bucket hat, not my wig, even though my wig matched my hair perfectly. But when my hair came in almost totally gray with only a little bit of brown (instead of the red-brown it had been), I had my hairdresser color it. The first dye job was probably 6 months after my last chemo and about 2 or 3 months after I quit wearing hats or my wig. It helped, but it didn't cover very well. I had a second dye job 6 weeks later which covered very well, and I'm going back for a cut and color. I waited to dye it the first time because it was so short, it didn't seem worth it. But my oncologist told me I could dye it as soon as there was enough there to dye.

kamaha

My hair straightened out as it got longer (and heavier). It was always naturally on the darker side, but I had been blond for several years, so a few months after I stopped wearing the wig, when it was still short, I had it highlighted. It took about a year to grow significantly, but only about 6 months to get a little weight and straighten out to the point where it stopped feeling like a Brillo pad!

RedBird, I think you should do whatever makes you feel good about yourself. As my social worker said, "if that's your coping mechanism, then use it!" When people who didn't know about my situation saw me with dark short hair and said "oh you got your hair cut!" I just smiled and said yes. As far as I was concerned, if they didn't know already, they didn't need to know.

Nushka

THE SHOCK OF THE NEW — YOUR HAIR, FOR BETTER AND FOR WORSE

Hard as it is to believe when you're going through chemo, happily at a certain point your hair does grow back. But all that gray and those quirky curls that seem to defy gravity! For me, I didn't just gain a new head of hair—I also gained an array of hair thickeners, glisteners, and pomades meant to tame my outer wild child.

"My hair came back great. It is curly and very thick. I actually like it better, though I could have done without the whole experience."

Traveler

I had very straight hair and mine came back very curly. It always was thick and it still is, thank goodness. People have told me that usually the curls relax after 6 months to a year. I've had hair for 6 months now and it's still extremely curly. I have to laugh about it, though. Lots of people thought I was so glad to have hair again that I got a perm!

kamaha

My head hair grew back the same except my widow's peak never returned. I have *no* underarm or leg hair, and very little hair on my um, private area. (I hear that the Hollywood babes are paying big bucks to get waxes that resemble my "chemo baldness.")

Stillhere

THE SOUTH POLE: LOSING HAIR *THERE*

In this three-way conversation the "unmentionable" is finally mentioned.

The worst part of losing hair was when I lost my pubic hair. Going to the bathroom, dropping your drawers and seeing more hair stuck to your panties than your skin was awful. We all talk about hair on our heads, underarms, and legs, and no support group I've been in has anyone mentioned losing their pubic hair, except once and that was very briefly.

KeyWoman

Dear KeyWoman,

I too was so shocked when my pubic hair came out in my panties. I too found that it is never talked about. I'm shocked! This is an important area to most people, too. If the doctor (male) didn't want to tell me, why in the world didn't his female nurse? I lost my eyebrows but not my lashes, and not the hair on my legs, but underarm hair went with the rest.

googie

Yea, losing the pubes was odd, made me feel weird, unfeminine. It was a shock that first time I went to the bathroom, pulled down my pants and there was a bunch. Somehow I did not expect that. That was the longest to grow back as well. I think because of the chemo, *pause*, perhaps.

RC

I was rather disturbed that one sensual and sexual body part was routinely discussed, a breast, yet pubic hair was passed over. I think it should be discussed, especially since so many women have problems with sex during and after treatment. It's okay to talk about vaginal dryness, but not the loss of pubic hair? That just doesn't make sense.

RC, I had this odd feeling of part of me reverting to childhood when I lost my pubic hair. The feeling was particularly strong when I would look at myself in the mirror after a shower—half of my chest flat and a pre-pubescent "nether region."

KeyWoman

Losing pubic hair was weird and sometimes I'd get cold and think perhaps I forgot to wear a panty.

Kgadi

Kgadi lives in South Africa.

I laughed when my pubic hair started falling out. I knew it could/would happen, but my husband thought it was sexy that I was all smooth.

Polish Princess

CHAPTER THREE

Feelings: A Kitchen Sink of Emotion

"A good friend who is also a survivor told me it was alright to have a bad day without feeling like you were being a bad patient."

beachbooks

This entire book could have been filled with entries about the feelings and physical changes that a diagnosis of breast cancer causes. The feelings we have from the time we are first diagnosed through treatment and recovery are like the proverbial "kitchen sink"—there's a little bit of everything here, with the words piling up as the women heap on story after story. And very few of these feelings happen in a vacuum: so many women react to their healthy friends or to the importance the media places on big breasts and cleavage. Questions such as "why me?" occur, but less than you might think. More than any one thing, the women react to the overall "before and after" impact on their lives. The woman who writes "I am sad I will never again experience feeling truly carefree" seems to be speaking for all of them.

If you've ever assumed that you're the only one who's ever felt anger or jealousy, or that a dark cloud is hovering just over your head, read on. Read about the many topics covered here in numbing honesty:

anger, fear masked as anger, blame, "breast cancer hell," control, depression, family and friendship, fatigue that's both physical and an emotional malaise, jealousy, loneliness, the "new" normal, and sadness. Although I was raised never to say the word hate, *I've included an entire section called "things I hate most," wherein women tick off things large and small that give them no end of agita. But all is not doom and gloom, and so this chapter ends on a positive note: coping, the benefits of yoga or exercise, and writing. And where do I see myself? In every single category. At one time or another, I've had all of these feelings, though not in equal measure.*

ANGER

You might think that anger only begets more anger, but it's not true—the kettle that whistles and the smokestack that blows off steam are about release, and sometimes that's the healthiest act a woman can do.

When I first got the diagnosis, I felt as if life kicked me in the teeth and I wondered what I did to deserve a cancer diagnosis. I went through a divorce nine months earlier to end a 27-year very unhappy marriage. Going through divorce was like being hit by a bus; getting a cancer diagnosis was like being run over by a freight train.

Carole

I cried all the tears I have when my sister became ill. Now my main emotional outlet is anger, and I'm a complainer. I tell my friends upfront: I'm going to complain about the pain, the weakness, the fear, the anxiety, the mounting housework because putting it "out there" reduces it.

Cath

I see a lot of "thankful" and "blessed" feelings expressed. But what about anger? I'm one who wrote that I believe everything happens for a reason, etc. But I also believe that deep down inside I have a lot of anger that my sane and rational exterior won't let me reveal. I suspect that I have harbored a lot of anger for *years* about my dad's cancer. It changed our family life and robbed us of our "normalcy." I was 15. Again at 46 it came to take some more from me. As stoic and accepting as I may seem, I believe there is one *angry* part of me.

scrapper

Sometimes I feel like people worry that I'm "fragile" and I hate that.

ginadc

I did have a rather heated argument (about visiting my brother who is in jail) with my parents and blurted out that I fear dying and orphaning my child, that I am angry with everyone who says "you are so strong, you'll get through this too" as if I were having a tooth pulled, etc. Now, not only don't we talk about my brother, my parents coddle me, not wanting to set off the time bomb again.

jennie

Anger!!!! Yes! I am very, very angry, even now, 18 months later. I resent the fact that I have spent my life watching my diet, exercising, not smoking or drinking, doing the right things, being a "good" girl. I have friends who smoke, drink, work too hard, don't exercise, etc., yet I am the one who got breast cancer. I do not feel thankful or blessed or grateful or any of those things. I am *angry*! And then when I think about the anger and how fruitless and self-defeating it is, I get angry at me for wasting my time being angry. Then I get depressed. Then I get angry because I am depressed. It is a vicious cycle.

We mostly aren't allowed to talk about the anger, particularly if we are done with treatment because we are supposed to be well and go on with our lives and forget that "bad stuff." I don't talk about the anger; most people don't even understand.

Nett

I don't think I was angry for "getting" cancer. I'm mostly angry about what it's done to certain aspects of my life. It made my husband distant. He couldn't really cope so went off on his own to cope in bars and a beer glass. We've never really recovered from this period of time. It broke down my trust of him and I can't seem to get it back. Our marriage was a struggle even up to that point, but it definitely was more challenging after my diagnoses.

I'm angry that it's brought my mortality so close. Most friends I have don't give death a second thought. That used to be me. I have become short-tempered, impatient, and ultimately my body shuts down and I sleep a lot.

Sara C

I myself do get angry when someone tells me that I don't look sick. "Look sick"—what does that mean anyway?

NMRose

The anger subject seems to just wax and wane with me. I guess that we (breast cancer survivors) just see it as *totally* unfair to have to experience this thing that cannot be understood by those who have *not* experienced it. I just try to accept that it may be overload for other people, even though it does hurt terribly. I say this because being a long-term survivor has made me see how it even affects my husband, children, siblings, etc. It's like we (as survivors) have to face it always, but others (no matter how close) think that they will preserve their selves from hurt or something by being distant.

I'm a 16-year survivor, recurred at 10 years, cancer-free again (hopefully), yet I am experiencing a great deal of anger right now. It's just there! A lot of it is about the way others treat me—without concern for what I experience now because of the cancer and its treatment. Even my dear husband, who has always been there, seems to understand less now than ever and he has "seen" it all, but he has not "experienced" it or its repercussions himself, thus *cannot* really understand.

> AmyT.16 yrsurvivor

Most of me says that I have no right to be angry, after all I have been so richly blessed in so many ways. But that small, hostile, immature person inside wants to lie on the ground, beat my heels on the floor, and screech "It's not fair!" at the top of my lungs. Do you think that will go away, or do you think I can at least tie her up and put her back in her closet?

> webfoot45

I don't think the anger ever truly goes away, it just goes into hiding only to come out when it is triggered by something or someone. I was at a barbecue last night and a woman (unaware of my situation) there was commenting on how her boobs are beginning to droop. Could you imagine only having *that* to worry about! Ugh! Now my anger just came out of the closet! See how easy that was????

> reginabu

I am angry as I just found out another friend has died from this ** disease. She was diagnosed after me by two years and is gone already.

> west coast woman

Anger at your doctor

It wasn't until I was writing an e-mail to someone, talking about my old oncologist, that I realized I am still very angry with her. I complained for almost three years and every time she would just pooh-pooh my complaints and say I had done something to cause the pain, like pulling a muscle or strained something. Then when it got to the point that I told her I could no longer stand it, she told me I can order a bone scan if it will make me happy and added that she was sure it wouldn't show anything. *Make me happy!* Yeah right, I was really happy to have her call and say, "Sorry, it looks like the cancer is back."

I do get angry when I think about the fact that I was going for my checkups and thought I was doing everything I needed to be doing and I went from having a tumor so small that it really wasn't even a stage to Stage IV. I was so naive that I really didn't ever think it would come back. When they told me I was Stage IV, I asked how many stages are there? When I found out I didn't have another stage to go to, the wind sure got knocked out of my sails. That was 6 years ago and I really think I am doing well, and I feel good. Angry? You bet I am.

Marybe

Anger is different when you're young

Now having been on both sides of the standard age cutoff "under 40," I feel that how and what we experience differs. Anger is one such feeling.

I've read that your chance of recurrence goes down the longer you have been cancer-free. But maybe these statistics were with older women; maybe they were already dead 10 or 15 years out from old age! Oh, see, now I feel better: I'm getting angry about these statistics that are probably wrong. I guess I do get angry . . . and afraid!

Lsurvivor

Anger and fear are so close together: Sometimes I am scared, and then I get angry that I'm scared! I think both have a healthy place in our healing. The problem is when one or the other takes over.

webfoot45

Webfoot45, this is my first experience with discussing my cancer with others in 10 years. I'll call it a support group, because I feel comfort in your responses. Just knowing I'm not the only one who feels this way and was diagnosed at a young age has helped me. When I was first diagnosed I went to a support group, but I was by far the youngest person there and it upset me more than it helped. I'm so grateful for the "40 and under" group,* I can't tell you. Before this, I was the only person I know who had breast cancer under 55!

survivor

*In the online project, younger women had the option to be in groups with other women under the age of forty.

BEING NUMERO UNO: PUTTING YOURSELF FIRST

"Don't ever apologize for your feelings."
jennagram

I would be a liar if I claimed I wasn't angry. I guess it falls under the "Life Isn't Fair" category. My biggest anger moments have come out over the weirdest things. For some reason during radiation it infuriated me that the techs would draw on me with markers for positioning the treatments. I understood the logic, but as I told them, it made me feel like a billboard that anyone could write graffiti on. I asked for and received the little tattoos for that purpose, but still they sometimes drew on me. One day the radiation oncologist did so, and I really lost it. I cried and yelled at them all! Fortunately they knew anger was part of the bargain and heard me out.

There are still days when I am very angry I have cancer, but now I ask myself why I think I'm special that I wouldn't have *something* I had to deal with. It helps keep the whole thing in perspective.

Lizzi

The anger is a natural part of the journey. The frustration of not being able to do what I was accustomed to doing was driving me bananas. I have always been that person who could go, go, go and still be bubbly and happy. When the fatigue hit me in a big way that put a big bump in the way I did things. I am one of those people that always takes care of the other guy first. Now I am in counseling. I really didn't think I needed it, but was encouraged by my family to go. I remember one of the first things the therapist said to me was that it was okay to be angry and frustrated. I had been through a lot. I needed to mourn the loss that cancer had thrown into my lap. I had never thought of mourning as being part of this process. I am learning to accept and to express what I want. Like my counselor said, Linda, you make sure everyone else is okay with this, but you have not done the same for you. You need to be first on that list. The others will take your lead.

Linda

When breast cancer hits you, you have to do what's best for you; you become Number 1.

jennagram

Anger at those who should know better

I felt guilty for having these thoughts: I am resentful because the people that I thought would be there for me were not. Sometimes, I just want to have a pity party, but only for a *moment.*

ladycmj2004

Ladycmj2004, I have found that most people are there for you in the beginning. After you have survived the surgery and the treatments they seem to think that everything is okay. They don't realize that surviving is an everyday event for someone who has had breast cancer. You will find that people really don't want to know the details. But I have found that family members are the most difficult to understand because they should know more than most what you are going through. My sister-in-law made the statement that she had not been around anyone with cancer and didn't know what to expect. She lives 125 miles from us and when I went through all of it she wasn't there to see. In her mind I survived, kind of like taking an aspirin for a headache so everything was right with the world. People just don't get it.

Jackjoy

Things that really piss me off are the people who were so damned concerned in the "beginning." Cards came in often. And phone calls, too. But when I really needed those people when my husband walked out on me and I had no money, where were they??? Nowhere to be found. If you are going to be a friend, be a friend for the entirety. Don't just "be there" for the initial onslaught as we all know that this disease is never ending.

In my case, having been a daughter-in-law and a sister-in-law for 27 years, now I hear from only one of the 5 "family" members involved. Go figure. The friends? Well, I evidently had friends who were superficial as they have not been there either. Again, go figure. There. I am done being pissed.

Ladyblue930

Walk a mile in *our* shoes

Sometimes I'm still furiously angry at being disfigured by this disease. I'm really mad that I had to go through menopause so young. Long-term side effects make me crazy. I know that it could have been much worse and of *course* I'm grateful to be here, grateful I had good doctors, etc. But no *way* am I going to be glad that I've been mutilated, poisoned, and aged 15 years in the last year.

Agent99

I've been poisoned, fried, cut up, and turned loose, and I feel very ill-prepared to cope. Things I trusted are gone. What has really knocked the props out from under me is the realization that nothing will ever be the same. I can't trust in my good health anymore, can't trust that continuing health issues won't take my job away. I feel vulnerable and exposed, and I hate it! Right now I feel very, very angry about the whole thing, and I never really had anger until now. I'm not even sure who or what I'm angry at, just the stupid cancer I guess.

Ro

You sound so much like me.

Msnegs

Chemotherapy was difficult for me the first time. I got tired of people telling me how important it was to be positive. I had to bite my tongue not to say, "You come over and stick your head in my toilet and I'll go over to your house and be positive."

beachbooks

I have a friend that had a double mastectomy last year. Don't ask her about having breast cancer because she will take it off and show you, "this is what breast cancer looks like—any questions?"

Jackjoy

I didn't tell my business associates until I was almost done with treatment. I'm glad I waited because they asked too often and disbelieved my answers. The hardest part was when they would comment on how "nice" my new hairstyle was. Since I was going through an angry part with my emotions, I wanted to yank the wig off, throw it on the floor, and stamp on it with both feet while exclaiming, "It's not my hair."

butterfly2

Anger at secondhand smoke

The person that makes me angry at times is my husband. He smokes and doesn't take care of himself. I ask him all the time "How can you look at me and what I'm going through and not stop smoking?" I don't get it. Anyway, what makes me angry is the thought that our boys could lose me and then what if he gets sick and they have no one.

ally

I didn't feel angry toward people who were smoking but sometimes I did feel amazed! Here I'd be, sitting at Starbucks on the patio with my golden retriever, drinking a cup of tea, bald, no eyebrows, skin gray, horribly skinny, and someone would come light up right next to me. Finally one day I walked up to a guy who was smoking and said, "Look at me. Do you *really* want to go through this?" and we had an interesting conversation. It's so normal to think we're invincible. I was jealous of people who could feel that way.

Agent99

THE BLAME GAME—WHY ME?

Did you ever blame yourself for "getting" cancer? Did you regret things you had done that may have "caused" you to get the disease? For example, my husband and I both immediately said it was our fault because I stayed on birth control pills for too long. Then I thought it was probably my fault because I had my first child when I was over 31 years old. I never smoked, etc. But these are both risk factors that I had "ignored." I found myself looking at the microwave oven as a possible offender—maybe it was nuking my breasts! I thought about all the chemicals that they put on the soccer field grass and how many soccer games I had sat through with my kids. It makes you crazy!

junebug

Even though I do not want to wish this disease on my worst enemy I do have a problem with Y-me!! I have no history of breast cancer in my family and have taken pretty good care of myself, exercise, and eat right. Some days I want things to go back to the way they were before breast cancer and be oblivious to the medical realities each of us has faced.

    rainbow

I look at people who abuse their bodies and wonder why I am going through this and not them. I have learned to control my anger and each day it gets easier.

    Doreen

I did not have too much trouble with Y-me because of my age—61 now, 58 when diagnosed with IBC. I have known others with cancer—some living, some deceased. I had come to view cancer as a very democratic disease: princes, paupers, presidents, and movie stars are not immune. At my age, acquaintances are beginning to get diseases like ALS, early dementia, Alzheimer's, crippling rheumatoid arthritis. Cancer takes its place in line behind most of those diagnoses, at least in my view.

    mountainmomma

Why me? Well, why not me? I'm not any more or less special than anyone else. If I had to make a choice between having this or someone else having this, I would certainly take it for myself.

    zoochild

I feel the same way. I was shocked one day when a group of friends were together. My sister was there and she said "why not me?" I had never thought of that; she has all these feelings and pain because I got stuck with this and she didn't. I tell her I'd rather it be me than anyone else in my family. I think it is easier to deal with it happening to me than the helpless feeling if it were another of my loved ones.

    ally

I think asking "Why me?" is a natural thought which is why I was surprised that I never asked it. I can only conclude that when you have a family history, you almost expect your turn to come, so the question seems answered.

> Juneboomer

Juneboomer learned that both she and her daughter are BRCA2 positive.

There's just a trace of gallows humor here!

Okay, you're going to think this is *completely* crazy, but . . . I smoked for sixteen years (and quit cold turkey, two weeks after meeting my husband). When I was diagnosed with breast cancer two years later, I assumed the smoking had something to do with it. The doctors, however, kept telling me that was impossible. I was sad that I had cancer, and I was angry that it was for no reason. Somehow, if it had been my own fault, it'd make more sense.

At this point, I have a social cigarette every once in a while. I figure if God's going to give me lung cancer on top of breast cancer, he *really* wants me dead. I told you that you'd think I was crazy.

> alleeum

Alleeum,

That is the funniest thing I have read!! I laughed so hard. I too quit smoking 2 years before I found my lump. I often feel angry because for the first time in my life I really started to get it together "healthwise." I quit smoking, was running, doing some kick boxing, and eating sooo healthy! I never looked or felt better and then bam! *Cancer.* Especially when people tell me about certain things to eat and exercise now that I've had a cancer diagnosis, I want to scream, "It doesn't matter, I WAS doing all that and still got cancer anyway!!!"

> Irish

"BREAST CANCER HELL"

Today, it seems, I am having another meltdown—usually happens once every month or so. After 17 months, I no longer experience the overwhelming fear that was with me 24 hours a day. I have, for some time now, come to a place where I am moving forward, trying to accept my new limitations and making the best of all that I do have. But on days like today, the antidepressant isn't quite working. I feel sad and I just so much want to be my old self again. I wouldn't mind having the knowledge I've picked up about myself and others, but I want to physically feel good. I don't want this incessant joint pain. I don't want to be 4 sizes larger. I don't want to see my scalp through my hair. I want to have hot, sweaty sex without the aides and the discomfort. I want my life back! I don't want to be an old woman at 54. Whaa, whaa, whaa. It's a one-person pity party. I'm not looking for more pity for, as you can see, I am experiencing no shortage. What I'd like to know is if any of you periodically share this negative exercise?

   San

San,

   You are not alone. I have those meltdowns too. But I share them with my friends and coworkers and it helps. I am lucky to have a very dear friend who would call me every other day when I was going through chemo and let me cry to her. We work together and I still cry on her shoulder when I need to. However, I no longer watch sad movies or watch the negative news on TV.

   Stillhealing

> "I found that a weekly rage and cry fest is good for the soul."
>
>   Sue

San,

I know exactly what you mean about meltdowns. I have had my share of those "pity days" as well. I too can sometimes go for weeks feeling great, and not letting anything get me down, but then I'll see or hear something that reminds me of all my trials and tribulations, that we have all shared to some degree, and I am in that "place" again, that mindset, back in time to "Breast Cancer Hell," where everything bothers or concerns me, and makes me fearful even to breathe. I also feel that it is better to stay away from sad TV shows, movies, news, etc.

I would venture to add though that if you listed the benefits, since you first became aware of breast cancer, they would outweigh the negatives. Even the small things that did not seem that important two years ago are magnified for me, and they would have been insignificant then. My, how time and a major illness changes us all!!

carolecare

CONTROL

Perhaps the most difficult thing for me in my journey was letting go of something over which I have no control. I was making myself crazy by second-guessing myself on everything and worrying that my decisions were the wrong ones. I think you must be an informed participant in your treatment and recovery, but once you have made your decisions, you have to put your faith in your doctors and let go and give it to God.

Mollynick

I know for me when I thought I had early stage breast cancer it was easier to cope; there were established protocols for treatment. But once I knew I was Stage IV, that was when I felt a complete loss of control, and it almost made me collapse.

Susie

I thought I was finally in control of my life when I was diagnosed with IBC. I explained to my sister this way: if I am going anywhere I need a map and then I don't worry because I know the next sign to look for. With IBC there was no map and I felt totally lost and it stressed me to the point that I was so afraid I was going in the wrong direction. What I'm getting at is that I had to get my map so I knew what I was doing and getting to the end of my journey. Chemo was my first stop, then MRM, then radiation, and now I'm on tamoxifen. My stress level decreased as soon as I knew what my treatments were and where I was headed.

lilybelle2

DEPRESSION, THE LETDOWN OF GETTING THROUGH THE WORST OF IT

After I was diagnosed I got on the treatment treadmill and I was exposed to a lot of people who were supportive and understanding of what I was going through. The doctors and nurses were wonderful. When it was all over, that support stopped. I also had the aftereffects of the treatment to deal with, the menopause, the changes in my physical appearance, and the uncertainty of cure. It took a while for me to get myself together. I might have looked okay on the outside but on the inside I was an insecure, raging mass of nerves. I started to take an antidepressant for the hot flashes. I still take it and it helped me. I think some depression is normal after what we go through.

MJ

Nice to hear that I am not the only one who was depressed after the treatment ended. The day I went to my last radiation treatment I cried when I left. I think we are so caught up in accepting our cancer and taking care of it with surgery, chemo, and radiation that when it's all over we don't know what to do. We wonder if everything we did "worked" the way it was supposed to and will we really be okay.

Polish Princess

Frankly, I'm scared to death. I'm 52, single, and self-supporting. I worked throughout treatment because there was no choice. I'm exhausted, and I'm terrified I'm not going to get well enough fast enough to hang on. My "significant other" has been back-pedaling as fast as he can to get out of the whole situation. This situation is probably adding to my depression. I feel like I survived treatment, but it remains to be seen how well I'm going to survive the overall experience of having cancer.

Ro

> "When you stop doing active things, that's when the depression and fear will start."
>
> JoAnn

It was a long time before I got angry, a matter of months in fact. I had been told so often that anger was wrong that I kind of put it away and refused to feel angry. As a result I think I suffered more depression.

Susie

FAMILIES AND FRIENDS: ANYBODY HOME??

It's one of life's oxymorons that emotional pileups tend to occur with people we're closest to—our family and dearest friends.

The one thing that sure bothers me more since diagnosis and treatment, and living with the recurrence stats, is family members that can be so hateful and greedy. Those that never pitched in with any of the trips to the hospital, caregiving of our families or other relatives and our parents, ask stupid questions about your plans if you don't make it, and criticize us behind our backs in just the other room. You learn who your real friends are, and blood is not thicker than water.

cow22girl

Oh, cow22girl, you've hit another nerve. My family was so concerned when I moved to the "big city"—said I didn't have any "real family" here, and that I'd regret it. Well, let me tell you who *was* here for me. My "real family" was too busy, uninterested, whatever, and I found out, maybe for the first time through my cancer, who my "family" was. I found that DNA makes no difference when defining "sister." And I will be forever grateful to them. To all of my *real* family (no DNA), who made meals, called every day, sent flowers, took me to the hospital at 5 AM, cried with me—whatever I needed—no amount of thanks will do. Blood is truly not thicker than water.

    mme jbc

When I think of emotions at this time (almost 6 years from diagnosis), I think that I have been emotionally hurt and confused over the fact some very important people in my life such as family and friends have not wanted to share this journey with me. They have acted, from the beginning, as if I never had breast cancer. Then, there were people in my life, those I least expected, who were there for me 200 percent. They still are. Even today, the others do not even want to hear the word "cancer" mentioned. Most have not said so, but I know so. I tell myself that I must understand and respect the feelings of others, but I would like to share this part of my life with siblings and close friends. It exists. It is an important fact in my life. Deep down, I know most care, but why have they chosen not to let me know it?

    Flower

Recognizing toxic people in my life and minimizing contact with them has been a means to protect myself. And the fact that I feel no loss confirms that they really weren't important to my life.

    Raesinthesun

I was talking with a friend of mine (at least I thought she was my friend) and telling her I was thinking about getting reconstruction and she had the nerve to tell me that she didn't think it was "fair" for my insurance to pay for my reconstruction. I asked her why and she told me that her insurance wouldn't pay for her to have a breast reduction back when she was in high school and it's like the same thing, right? She has a very small dimple in her breast and I'm missing half my chest.

joules112

My best friend (who is also single) and I were talking on the phone a couple of weeks ago. Mind you, she was there with me through almost the entire experience. She had commented how it has been so long since she has had sex and we should go out and find a couple of boys to play around with (half-jokingly, I think). My response to her was, "I can't do that anymore" and she said something real dumb like "How come?" I explained to her then that I can never just jump into bed with a man again because I would have to have had told him about my breast cancer experience before we even think about that. I then said, "I may look good with clothes on and you may not be able to tell, but that all changes when I take my clothes off." She then says, "Oh, are the scars that bad?" I remember thinking during my 2nd year that I wish there was a planet I could go to with only breast cancer survivors!

reginabu

Sometimes you lose even the most important friendships

I suspect this story will resonate for some readers.

Yes, I lost many friendships because of the cancer. There were two in particular that were extremely important to me, my two best friends. Both of them I knew for ten years. One of them I tried to call but she never called back so finally I left a message and sent an e-mail with more details. The second was my very best friend in all the world.

And I know people say she couldn't have been such a great best friend if she just disappeared. But it isn't that simple. We did get in a fight, and I asked her to give me some space and time. Since I was diagnosed I've never seen her again.

I have made new friendships of course, but none were like the friendship of the second woman I speak of—she was one of those friends that come along once in a lifetime and you just *know* each other in and out. She was more like a sister than a best friend. We had the same name and I looked kind of like her sisters. Her mom was my mom away from home. I haven't seen any of her family again. It's still devastating to me as nothing has replaced it. There is no one I can call every day, whenever I want, and talk about anything like I could with her.

pineapplejoey

Pineapplejoey,

I too have lost my "best friend." We've been friends since elementary school (over 24 years). I could say "our lives have taken different directions" or some other B$ but the truth is, I am hurt. I was there when her life was falling apart but I should have known when I told her my diagnosis and she responded "Wow. It is always some drama thing with you." As if I manifested cancer. I love her and I miss her but this says far more about her than it ever will about me.

Hang in there, sister!

jennie

FATIGUE

Fatigue before breast cancer and fatigue because of breast cancer are about as different as a cough and a hiccup. The fatigue that comes from chemotherapy, or from surgery, from radiation, from just dealing with the whole thing emotionally or physically is H-U-G-E. You are, as one woman writes with simple precision,

"Always tired." I can recall days when I would crawl into bed—not flop, not climb, but crawl—and sink into the bedcovers. Mornings when I couldn't rise, afternoons when I desired rest, evenings when I was lethargy personified. Only my cat found all this lying about fun, *seizing upon it as an opportunity to have round-the-clock nap time with me.*

Wanting to exercise is quite different from actually getting yourself to take a walk or go to the gym. Wanting to lose the weight you've gained because of fatigue and actually being able to do so is doubly defeating. Feelings of fatigue linger well past the time of actual treatment and become one of the silent hurdles women have to contend with.

Always tired. I can sleep 8 hours, 10 hours, whatever, and still want to take a nap a couple of hours after I am awake. I also find that I would love to take a nap just about every afternoon. I do have a low thyroid, but have been on medicine for about 3 years now for that. In my heart I believe this is all from the chemo as prior to that I was fine; maybe it is a combination, maybe stress. I am overweight, thank-you chemo and tamoxifen, a total of 60 pounds gained, and I know that is some of it.

Autumn

"There are definite peaks and valleys in the energy cycle, so take advantage of the high energy times and learn to listen to your body when it is time to slow down."

junebug

I notice I have "chemo" days. Days when I feel the old, familiar, just can't lift my head kind of tired. They don't come often but when they do I am just wiped out. I also have found it hard to get back into shape, mostly because once you have lost all muscle tone from being so out of action it is very hard to build it back up again.

Mostly it is just hard to get into the groove of a regular exercise schedule.

Sallie

I am four years after treatment and the fatigue has lessened quite a bit. I cannot keep up the pace I once did, working full time, housework, yard work, wife, mother, volunteering, etc. But I don't know if that is age or the aftereffects or both. I try to pick and choose what I can do and learned to say "no" to myself and to others (and I do mean "learned" because it takes practice and I still say "yes" from time to time when I should say no). Eating right, getting a bit of exercise (particularly walking because it is relaxing and meditative as well as good for you), and getting enough sleep are all important for the energy.

junebug

I am always exhausted. I wonder how long it will be until I feel "normal" again. No matter what I do, my level of energy is so limited . . . going shopping, socializing, working (home and elsewhere), I always feel tired. I don't say anything, but I am certain that the people in my life are aware of the change in my activities. I really just want to feel healthy again.

Jacquie

I, too, feel constantly fatigued. My joints ache and I am definitely not as spry as I used to be. I always blame the tamoxifen or the fact that I have a 2-year-old. These are symptoms I can live with though. I feel very fortunate to be alive so I rarely complain.

Lauren

And then there's the exception to every "rule"

I am about eight weeks out from radiation which followed about 10 months of chemo. I feel better than I think I have felt in my entire adult life. I'm sleeping better than I have in several years. I am work-ing full time and raising a three-year-old and enjoying long summer days in Alaska. I attribute all this to daily 45-minute walks and an organic whole foods diet. No sugar, including fruit sugars, and very low carbs. I eat lots of fish, chicken, tofu, and lots of veggies. I get lots of protein. I eat very little processed foods. It has been so long since I've had sugar that the three pints of Ben & Jerry's brought for dessert and left in my freezer last night aren't even tempting!

Helen

JEALOUSY AND ENVY

I sometimes have a hard time relating to my friends who have not experienced cancer. I am envious of people who have not gone through this devastating experience.

panthergirl

I am not envious of people who have not had cancer nor would I wish it on anyone, not even my worst enemy. I just think some of us get it and some of us don't. It's not from anything we did and we weren't singled out, we just had the misfortune of getting it. One thing I have found is that if you look around, you can always find someone who is in worse shape than you are.

Marybe

My sister-in-law is going to get married at the end of the summer. I look at her and listen to her talk about how easily she will get pregnant and how confident she is in her health and I seethe with jealousy. Sometimes I listen to my friends talk about their babies and their new pregnancies and all the nice stuff that is going on in their lives and I have to bite my tongue to stop from ruining their happiness with my anger.

Max's Mommy

Envious of other women and their breasts

Being 5 weeks post-op from the second mastectomy, I found myself envious of other women's breasts, but only when they flaunt them and reveal a lot of cleavage. I have to screen what I am watching on TV as there's so much of that in movies (love scenes), music videos, etc., that it triggers so much sadness I just break down crying and sobbing. I also notice other women's breasts a lot—not in a sexual way of course, but I guess in an envious way, as a woman who can't have children would notice all the other women who are pregnant, or just had a freshly hatched baby.

Big Red

> "I'm grateful to be here but I'd prefer to be here whole."
>
> hotflash

When I first started down the reconstruction road I was looking forward to my new chest. I was going to be bigger, more perky, with new nipples. Now that I am at the end of reconstruction and we've reconstructed all that can be reconstructed, I find myself more jealous than ever of women who still have their own breasts, especially nipples. I find myself staring at other women's chests, wondering if they know how lucky they are to still have their breasts. There are still those dark moments, those sad moments, when I envy those with real nipples. I miss mine, the way they looked, the sensation in them. To know I'll never have that again. Just isn't fair. Not at 32, not at any age.

Squirrel

LONELINESS

People speak of being "puffed up with pride"; well, loneliness can fill you up, too.

It's hard to keep educating people we know and love, but the alternative is to feel like there's a huge chasm (instead of just an occasional chasm) between you and anyone who hasn't had this experience. Which is ultimately a very lonely way to live . . .

oceanwalker

Oceanwalker, you have touched a nerve that I feel fairly often, although overall I have a wonderful, happy life with many family and friends. Loneliness—it is an emotion I was not really familiar with until I was diagnosed and it still makes me uncomfortable to admit that sometimes I feel lonely, even surrounded by those who care for me the most. I even feel it sometimes after I attend my breast cancer support group, because most of them do not have mets and can't really understand what it is like, or are terrified of getting mets themselves. This is when I often pray, just by myself, for help in continuing to make connections in my life. Funnily enough, the people who can make me feel the least lonely are my oldest friends from high school, who have all been very supportive and more in touch in the past three years than ever before, although we are all still very close.

songbird

Songbird, I think that's just part of the human condition, no? Like you, I think of my life as full and rich and happy (which was also true before breast cancer). But there are moments when I'm just in my own experience of fear or anxiety and it's just me, by myself, trying to work through it. I think it does help to talk with others who share similar experiences, and I'm guessing that when you talk with other women who've been diagnosed with mets you feel less lonely, and less like "the other." I really count on my friends who've been diagnosed with breast cancer—or whose lives have been affected by cancer—to help me get through some of those darker moments in which there seems to be such a huge rift between me and others who've never dealt with cancer.

oceanwalker

THE "NEW" NORMAL

Nearly every single woman in this book at one point or another made comments to the effect that when the obvious signs of her disease or treatment no longer showed those around her expected that she'd go "back" to being "normal." Guess again.

> "I want to just live and not always have to focus on the big picture and be responsible as a survivor!!"
>
> shari

What angers me most is that some of the very people who helped me survive this awful journey now assume it is all over and I am back to normal. I have a positive attitude and a good prognosis, but what happened to me is not going away and is still with me every day (how can you see scars like that and not think about it)!

Anonymous

I, too, get ticked at people when they just don't understand what we have truly endured. We are no longer normal . . . yeah, we are . . . just a *new* normal.

DonDonJac

I want to look and feel "normal" again. I guess that won't happen, but I am holding out hope. I do not want to wear my disease like a battle scar for all to see. I don't want to be a walking advertisement for breast cancer.

Jacquie

I was beginning to wonder about myself. I have been so strong throughout everything and now that I have had my final reconstruction (2 weeks ago) I am surprised that I am jumping at every ache and pain and wondering if it is just some sort of withdrawal or if I really should be so worried that it is coming back in another part of my body. I never expected to be feeling this way as I have so longed for it all to be over so I can be "back to normal."

ScaredSilly

I finished treatment 2 years ago and to this day I cannot find normal. At times, I go as I did before and all of a sudden it hits me: I had *cancer*!!!

graciela0107

Ladies, *normal* is only a cycle on the washing machine!!

Purplepassion

SADNESS AND SHAME

Sadness is heartbreaking. Period. Full stop.

> "I feel sad and I just so much want to be my old self again."
>
> San

It makes me angry when I tell people I am scared and they say to me "you will be fine!" How do they know whether or not I will be fine, whether or not I will die from breast cancer? What makes them think this somehow makes me feel better? I just want to hit them! But mostly I am just sad.

I am sad that so few people supported me throughout this journey.

I am sad no one visited me when I was in the hospital for 3 days for my mastectomy, not even my parents who live an hour away.

I am sad that my sister has never once even acknowledged my cancer (and I see her frequently).

I am sad about how much my relationships with my friends and family have changed.

I am sad no one ever came to my house to bring me a meal, to offer with house work or food shopping.

I am sad to have my vitality taken away from me at such a young age.

I am sad for my husband and what he has had to experience in the past 20 months, and what he continues to experience, and what he will have to experience in the future.

I am sad I will now never hold my own child in my arms.

I am sad about all the emotional pain that just doesn't seem to want to heal.

I am sad I will never again experience feeling truly carefree.

I am sad about how sad and scared and lonely I always feel.

Alix

"If I think of those I lost to this disease, I can cry for an hour. If I think of all those I have lost to cancer in general, I can cry for a lifetime."

Autumn

I had an odd experience last night. I just started seeing a therapist and she asked me to think about what makes me angry. I have been thinking about my sister who died due to incompetent care, anger at the treatments we have to go through, and anger at myself. I live in a small town and decided to walk to the grocery store still in some degree of pain from my bilateral mastectomy. When I arrived my thoughts took me back to my childhood and some of the psychologically abusive things my mother did to me and my siblings, and I started crying on the way home. I was trying to hold back my tears, remembering that Mom had always humiliated me by calling me a "crybaby"—even when I was very young—so I learned to hold back tears.

It made me realize I am not so much angry as hurt. And it's "safer" for me to be angry than sad. My anger is not going to change anything in my past. I have to face my sadness to move on to the next stage of my life.

I'm so inspired by the women here because I learned it's possible to be strong and sad at the same time.

Susie

If I think of those I lost to this disease, I can cry for an hour. If I think of all those I have lost to cancer in general, I can cry for a lifetime. As I write this, my eyes start to tear, for all those I have lost to cancer: numerous friends (17), some I met due to breast cancer, some were best friends (2), some were family (3), and one, my mother, although that was lung cancer, it is still *cancer*, and that word sucks!

Autumn

THINGS I HATE MOST

Anger is a feeling. Hate is a declaration.

1. I hate that I look ugly. I'm only 49.
2. I hate that my kids think I look funny. Tonight I was having

dinner and a little girl at another table looked over at me and said "hello"; she was so cute, about 3. Her dad leaned over and said "shhhh, don't stare" and then I felt like a freak for the rest of my dinner and couldn't wait to get out of there.

3. I hate that I don't feel like "me" anymore.
4. I hate that I might not live to see my kids grow up.
5. I hate that I could have passed it on to my daughter.
6. I hate that my sister might get this. My mom and her sister both had it; my aunt died from it.
7. I hate it when people share their friend of a friend's cancer story and that when you ask how the person is, they say "he/she died." What's the deal? I want to hear that they survived and are still here.
8. I hate that estrogen is what keeps women young but is now my #1 enemy.
9. I hate that they haven't found a cure.
10. I hate how I feel: numb and painful feet and hands from carboplatin and taxol.
11. I hate that I had an allergic reaction to the carboplatin and can no longer take it and have one less option to fight this horrible disease.
12. I hate that it spread to my liver.
13. I hate living in fear.

ally

I hate that I won't ever need a mammogram again.

Bonbon

I hate that I'm 42 and in menopause with hot flashes and a totally dried-out vagina.

I hate that I lost my beautiful hair and my new hair is black. *Black.* I'm supposed to be *blond.*

I hate of course that I lost my breast, which was a very nice breast.

I hate that no matter what I do I'll never ever have my body back to what it was.

I hate that I've become "wiser." I know, I know, that's really a good thing but I wasn't too unhappy thinking life could be great all the time.

I hate that my daughter had to go through watching me be so sick and that she had to be afraid I'd die.

I hate thinking I might have passed this on to her.

I hate that in most groups of breast cancer women I have to now add that of course, I'm grateful to be alive, blah, blah, blah. I think that should go without saying. I hate having to act like a good little cancer patient.

Agent99

I hate my body profile.

I hate that I think it will prevent me from ever attracting a man again.

I hate that I think it makes a difference.

Isurrender

Add the stupidity of some people and what they say, like: "How bad can it be? My mother had it and she's still alive." (Well, my mom didn't make it and now I have it.) How about, "Well, it's only hair!" (Did anyone shave their head in support of your hair loss?) The doctor who told me, "We'll watch, wait, and see what happens."

sibling rivalry

These women are all under the age of forty

What really pisses me off is:

1. Just because I have cancer all of a sudden I'm a magnet for all those people who want to share stories of friends of a friend's first cousin removed who lives in Timbuktu who died at 20 with

cancer less dangerous than mine. What's up with this? Does anyone care that hearing this can be upsetting to someone surviving cancer hearing all the time that people are dropping dead??

2. I really don't get those people who go to a cancer fundraiser and then go outside to smoke. Do they not think about those going in and out the door who have cancer or those who don't that have to inhale that stuff? Kill yourself but leave me out of it.

3. I really hate my implants. Yeah, they don't look horrible in a shirt, although I see every little flaw; they are hard, painful, and I hurt daily and yet these poor women do this daily to themselves to gain self-esteem? Go figure.

4. My eyebrows, eyelashes, and hair on my body still fall out. I got it back but it comes out as easy as wiping my face and to me it is a constant reminder of what I lost in the first place.

But most of all I *hate* that every time I get sick or don't feel well my poor kids begin to worry now because cancer put that fear in their hearts, and I know it will be a long time before they get past this and that breaks my heart.

Princess86

> "I hate being so tired that I long for my toddler's nap."
>
> Max's Mommy

I hate that having cancer has made me realize that bad things happen to good people. I used to be the first one to tell people that "it would be okay" and "not to worry." Now I find myself saying "Well, it's better to get it checked out sooner rather than later."

I hate having to use the phrase "Since I went through chemo (or surgeries/radiation/had cancer)" in my sentences about how my life has changed.

> LukesMom

I hate that in 5 months' time I can age an entire decade.

I hate that I scare small children in public places.

I hate that my 3½-year-old daughter panics when she sees me in pain.

I hate that at this moment there are women freaking out at just having heard their breast cancer diagnosis.

I hate that I may not learn anything from this experience.

> Mamaper

> "I hate that all of us had to go through this.
> It just isn't fair."
>
> atoth

I am angriest about two things:

First, that I may have passed on this F@*&'ing mutation (I'm BRCA1) to my daughter, who is 2½. There's a 50 percent chance that I have.

Second, that I may not be here to see her grow up.

> Stillhere

> "One thing that I really hate is that having
> breast cancer has changed how optimistic I
> used to be."
>
> LukesMom

I miss my eyebrows! I miss my hair and I hate wearing a wig in 90 degree heat. I hate that I start sweating like a horse and then my carefully applied eyebrows run down my face!

I hate wondering how future boyfriends will take this and whether I will have any sex drive and the wondering if I will ever find someone who can cope with a breast cancer survivor!

Daisy19

I hate that I *still* can't fill out a sexy nightgown, even after reconstruction. These things were supposed to look great—it was one of the only positive things (physically) about this experience. I had originally barely been a size A. So going to a C was supposed to make me look better. Little did I know they won't ever look like the real thing. Maybe my expectations were too high.

I hate that I did the "nipple" thing and it didn't work—one died and the other is going flush with the rest of my skin. Now they are just ugly scars.

I hate that my husband has to live the rest of his life without boobs. Will he be thinking of someone else's?? I know he loves me and we have an amazing marriage, but come on—he's a man! What man is just okay with no boobs the rest of their life???? Good thing he's in love with me, huh?

I hate that this thing could come back at any time, this horrible thing that could kill me, that could take me away from the man I was so fortunate to find to share my life with. This thing that could prevent me from having a baby. I ache at the thought.

Squirrel

Public enemy #1: the health insurance companies

Over the years in dealing with breast cancer, I had three different health insurance carriers. Each presented themselves as roadblocks in my care and treatment.

I would have to say I hate the f***ing insurance companies and how it seems like they screw us after all we have already gone through. Then we have to fight with them to be able to afford our meds or reconstruction.

bridgett

When it was time for me to have my nipple surgery the insurance company denied me saying it was cosmetic. I wrote back and told them if they could find me a definition or a picture of a breast without a nipple I might concede. I also spoke, of course, of the psychological impact no nipple would have and asked if they wanted to pay for counseling later. One little letter was all it took, but why was it necessary?!

hotflash

My insurance company was cooperative up until my nipple tattooing needed repeating (still faded too much). The insurance lady at my plastic surgeon's office told me I was at the mercy of my insurance company. No way, no how. My mercy comes from God alone. I wrote my plastic surgeon a letter saying just that. A few days later he zipped a letter off to United Healthcare quoting the federal laws, etc., which quickly prompted approval for the second tattooing.

Captiva96

COPING—YOGA, MEDITATION, THERAPY, DRAWING, AND WRITING

When all is said and done, let's end on a positive note.

> "Taking care of yourself is the most important priority."
>
> Smilie

Stress, do I ever understand that. I was lucky enough to have a support group and they were talking about a class in which you align your mind, body, and spirit. I made a decision that it was time to make a major change in my life and I signed up for the class. It was the start of a new chapter in my book of life. I found that things that weren't important weren't worth the effort to worry about them and that there is so much more out there. I reduced my stress to the point my boss asked me one day what I had done with the "real me." I set aside 30 minutes each day, without fail, for myself. I do some meditation and write down my feelings about whatever may have been a challenge or a wonderful thing that had happened during the day. I can't believe how different this small amount of time has changed my attitude.

siggy001

When I was diagnosed with breast cancer, I was devastated. I decided that I was going to give myself one day to cry, and then I was going to start to fight the cancer. On the way home from the diagnosis, I decided to go on a search to find items with positive messages and inspirational books. I shaved my head before the chemo/cancer took it. It made me feel very much in control. It made me feel powerful as if I was saying, it is my hair, and I will decide when it goes. I joined a meditation group, which met once a week. The calm and caring attitude of the people within the group was contagious. My husband and I meditated every morning and every evening. His support at each and every turn of my personal healing journey was truly overwhelming; he attended every aspect of my treatment. I exercised throughout my treatment, and I changed my eating habits. I get eight hours of sleep each night, which is not always easy. I continue to write in a journal. When I see my feelings on paper, they become easier to deal with. I have stopped worrying about things that I can't control.

To celebrate my first year of surviving, we adopted a puppy. Since then, we have adopted two more. We now have three dogs and one cat (we've had the cat for several years), so I get pet therapy each and every day. My pets always understand how I feel, and they are always willing to offer TLC.

Elaine

fear

"I think however you choose to deal with fear is
uniquely yours, like the cancer that grew inside
of you without your knowledge or permission.
Only you know how to move ahead."

DianaRmn

Even the most mentally healthy woman admits to having fear at some point while coping with breast cancer. Fear of losing your husband, fear of not being around to raise your children, fear of a recurrence, fear of losing your job, fear of losing your sexuality, fear of dying . . . this is a long list of very serious concerns. On the plus side are the many possible ways to address fear. I have been blessed with the sort of hardwiring that stares down fear. For some reason this is one rocky shoal I seem naturally able to navigate. But that doesn't mean I have never feared a premature death or a life pocked with illness. On more occasions than I care to admit I've feared a recurrence when I feel pain in some part of my body; if the fear-to-pain ratio increases or persists, then I call my doctor. I don't suffer alone, but to the contrary, I try to be proactive, to do something. That's how I am comforted. That said, I think fear is a natural emotion—tidal, lunar, and hormonal. Or to quote Sherlock Holmes, "It's elementary, my dear Watson."

"I think to have fear is to be human."

Lauren

FEAR OF NOT BEING THERE
FOR YOUR CHILDREN

I thought before I was diagnosed that I understood what fear meant. I truly didn't. Fear was waiting outside a doctor's room for test results knowing that a few sentences could end your life. Fear was looking into my children's eyes and hearts knowing that possibly the person who loved them most in the entire world might die.

Meta

"Friends periodically call in a panic if I've kept too low a profile, convinced something is wrong. I've learned to keep in contact with friends I don't see regularly."

Toni

Every now and then, when I least expect it, my biggest fear of leaving my husband alone with two kids to raise comes creeping into my head. My husband has been such a saint through all of this, but I fear he would really be so far out of his element if left alone to raise my daughter. I worry much more about her than my son because as hard as he may try my poor husband just cannot fashion a proper ponytail. I know that seems very trivial, but she is only 6 now. What would he do when she has her period?

ARSteach

> "What I fear most now is not living my life the way I choose."
>
> panthergirl

I had an attack of fear yesterday when my 5-year-old son's fish died. (It sounds a bit silly when I write it.) He knew it was sick for about a week. He knew that he was going to bury it when it died. He knew it was going to Fish Heaven. When I told him it had died he cried for an hour and a half before bedtime. Big tears rolled down his face. I am sure you all understand why this made me panic.

I gained comfort from my daughter who comforted him by putting her arms around him and said "just remember the happy times you had together." It made me smile.

Meta

FEAR OF RECURRENCE

In the beginning, I had my mom to talk to every day; she was going through her chemo for lung cancer. I lost mom almost 4 years ago, and now I find I have no one to talk to about the fear. My companion (domestic partner) is always supportive, but the words are, "Well, wait until you find out for sure." I agree I should, and I also know I can't. I get *scared*!! Bottom line, I am *afraid* it will come back some day. There have been nights I just lay there holding my dog; sometimes I feel she understands more than anyone else I could talk to, except of course you ladies here! I travel for my work often, and I wind up taking a stuffed animal with me that Jenn (domestic partner) gave me, and I hug that when thoughts sneak in at night. People try to say the right things, but they do not understand the fear.

Autumn

> "When I was treated shoddily by a breast cancer survivor, I realized that she was not an evil person, but that I was her worst nightmare."
>
> Toni

I too have fear that the cancer will return. Every time I get a new ache or pain I have myself convinced the cancer is coming back. I recently read a book about the law of attraction—how if we think negative thoughts we will surely attract them. So what I try to do is keep telling myself I am going to be cancer-free and to get my mind off the negative. I also try to get myself involved in something else so I don't think about it. This may sound stupid, but that's all I've got for now.

clk913

I am angry because having had cancer means to me that I am sentenced to a measure of fear for the rest of my life. Fear of every future mammogram. Fear that a headache that persists might really be something more. Fear that any vaginal bleeding might really mean a more serious problem. Fear of recurrence. I get most angry when I have this "fear" reaction that I cannot control.

junebug

TALKING WITH FATTY

Fatty was a wonderfully giving and spirited woman. After having conquered a very difficult life from childhood into her early adulthood, she writes of one remaining fear: the mortuary. The message couldn't be clearer.

My fear is that when I die I have to go to the mortuary. I am so afraid of that. I know it is irrational but there it is. I would like to stay at home until they bury me but it is usually so hot here* that I don't think it is allowed. I will have to check on that, but it does seem such a silly question to ask and such a silly fear.

fatty

Fatty was living in Cyprus.

Fatty, about a year ago I talked to the nun at my church about what was important for me when I died, what kind of a service I wanted. I quaked before I did this, thinking did I know what I was doing, and was this morbid. Funny thing is, it gave me peace just bringing issues in the open. And I'm relieved, because who knows when my mets will get out-of-hand, but then even if I get hit by that proverbial truck today when crossing the street, I am comfortable for having articulated my fears and for speaking the words "I will die." I laugh sometimes, because how could I think I wouldn't?

Fatty, it's a hard thing to embark on, but it's important to have a say in how we leave earth. I'm rooting for you and my prayers are with you.

Toni

Fatty, I'm rooting for you and my prayers are with you too. I want to let you know that you have touched my heart. I am slightly claustrophobic and the thought of being put in a box with no windows, no air—a coffin—frightens me. But I keep reminding myself that my soul cannot be boxed up, and that helps.

Mawsquaw

While I will go kicking and screaming, long ago I made arrangements for my earthly departure. It is a lot easier to get over that fear while you are healthy. I try to keep my checkups in perspective: if something new is found, I'll work with it.

jjensen

Hi All,

Thanks for your support. I will take your advice and talk to someone about this fear of the mortuary. It is so irrational as I will be dead and won't feel anything, will I? I am sorry, but I am not a believer in God as most of you seem to be. That makes death harder, as I believe when you're dead you're dead—no nice heaven to go to and meeting relatives and friends. I have not had an easy life; I seemed to get everything that was in the papers. I was sexually abused as a child from the age of 4 to 13. I had my daughter at 18 and was unmarried in the 1960s. It was not a pleasant experience as I got sent to a home which was horrible: it was run by the church and you all had to go and pray in the shed in the bottom of the garden; apart from that I remember a lot of scrubbing floors. The plan was that the church would take your babies and have them adopted, but that was not going to happen to me and I kidnapped my own baby. My first husband was a wife beater. My second lives in fantasy land and is a compulsive gambler. On the plus side I have a beautiful daughter who is generous, loving, kind, and with a smashing sense of humor, as well as 6 healthy grandchildren.

    fatty

Fatty, you touch me deeply and I want to say that I am sorry for all the pain you have endured in your life. You clearly have made a good life out of awful experiences. Bravo. I want to tell you that it is not so much your "irrational" fear of the mortuary, it is more what that mortuary represents: the ending of your relationships and leaving what you know and those you cherish. Enjoy your daughter and grandchildren to the fullest and don't let anyone tell you how to proceed with your life. The problem with fear is that it keeps you out of the present with our lives in the now. Follow your heart for you have wisdom. Of that I am most certain.

    Marcia

Fatty, my heart goes out to you. I do understand some of what you have gone through, since we have shared some similar experiences. I was also abused, sexually, from about 3 or 4 until about 13. Many of the choices I made as an adult were the result of those experiences. One thing I have learned over the years is that the things that were the most difficult for me to handle are the things that made me the strongest. It took me a lot of years to realize that, and to understand the connection between my adult behavior and the childhood sexual abuse. But I finally was able to say "no" to the people who were abusing me and learned that I can be victimized only for so long, and then I refuse to take it any longer. I'm getting better at setting boundaries so I don't have to be victimized or tolerate "abuse" before setting my foot down.

As far as your fears being irrational, aren't most fears, in some way or other? That doesn't make them any less fearful. It took a lot of courage to admit your fears; that same courage will help you work through them.

HopeNFaith

I am not the little girl or the young woman those things happened to, although I must say that having them happen I think marked me as a victim. The abuse made me feel that way and for a long time I did not like myself. That is not the case now. I think this has come with time and I think that breast cancer helped with that. After my recurrence there's no stopping me.*

fatty

*Fatty was from the U.K. and moved with her husband to Cyprus in 2003 in a bid to lead a gentler life following diagnoses in 1997 and again in 2003. She died in 2006.

HUSBANDS

My biggest fear is losing my husband. And in that I mean that he will die before me and leave me to cope with this on my own. I love him so dearly and he has been so incredibly supportive and strong through all of this that I truly would have collapsed on my own. I was 42 and he was 43 when we married. It is the first marriage for both of us. So having waited so long to find this terrific partner, I just don't want to have to do it without him.

Kellyk01

My husband is even older than I, part of that generation unable to open up with his emotions. However, after my recurrence and his own poor diagnosis, we have been able to talk and he has been far more cooperative than ever. When he was younger he was happier and less angry, was far more positive about everything. I don't expect him to make a U-turn, but things are more pleasant. Can you imagine cancer bringing you closer together?

jjensen

My husband and I have known each other since we were 15 years old and we're both 65 now. We've been married 33 years and he is a rock for me. He is frightened, too, and sometimes we cry together in our mutual fear. But for the most part, we hold on to each other for dear life, as it were. I lean on him more than he leans on me and sometimes wonder if I'm putting too much of a burden on him. Bless you all, ladies, I'm going to paint a gorgeous picture of a mountain lioness—my totem.

Annie Mac

CONQUERING FEAR

I fear hearing the words "your cancer is back" more then anything! I fear hearing "we see something on your mammogram and have to take more views." I fear these things but not one of them prevents me from moving forward with my life. My husband and I are in the process of adopting a baby from Korea, an exciting prospect that brings about a whole different level of fears. I want to be here to watch my baby grow into a young person. So for me fear is something to acknowledge and then move on because after all fear is just a feeling, not the sum total of who we are. Just as statistics are good to know but are not the definitions of who we are.

Hummingbird

"Fear was my motivating factor to do whatever it took to mitigate this disease."

jjensen

Here's an admission: when I wake up petrified (occasionally now) in the middle of the night, I hold one of my old stuffed animals and that helps more than anything else, since I won't wake up my husband to interrupt his sleep. I think when we are scared, we just want comfort first of all, since we know in our minds (if not our rapidly beating hearts) that we can't really get reassurance that works completely. If retreating to childhood comforts help, so be it.

songbird

"It seems that my coping mechanism has been to stay angry enough so that I don't have to acknowledge the fear. Does that make any sense?"

Anna Marie

When I was quite young, less than 10, my maternal aunt was dying of breast cancer. Having seen her bedridden at home and then hospitalized with tubes coming out of her body all over the place, I was terrified of breast cancer, or any illness for that matter. That was in the 1940s and cancer was a death sentence. My first diagnosis was 50 years later and I was determined to educate myself as well as I could about the diagnosis, prognosis, and courses of treatment. Fear was my motivating factor to do whatever it took to mitigate this disease. So I think fear can be positive. I am afraid of flying (instant death) and I let the fear paralyze me for so many years. I subjected my family to driving vacations. I rationalized that my kids needed me, their kids, etc. When it hit me that I am not indispensable, I gave myself permission to fly and thereby "go in peace." I am still fearful, but not ruled by my fears.

I think the issue of control also comes up here. We have a disease we cannot control; our doctors (or pilots in my case) and our disease have the control. While we can be educated consumers of medical services, we are sitting in the back seat. It is totally fearful to not be in charge of your body. But you can be a very good caretaker of your body and what happens to it.

jjensen

FEAR AS DENIAL

My youngest daughter, who was almost 18 at the time of my diagnosis, refused to talk about it, to go to the hospital, or have anything else to do with treatment. When the subject would come up, she would get angry. It was really hurtful until a psychologist pointed out that anger is almost always fear-based. The anger was usually easier to take than the seeming indifference. Yet she is the one who expressed her feelings, first by making a graphic print of a mastectomy surgery, and then by explaining that it was her way of dealing with everything.

HopeNFaith

My mother who is 83 was in denial: 3 of us were diagnosed last year with breast cancer and she was one of them. I believe that she just could not accept the fact that all of us were diagnosed in the same year. Her mother had died of breast cancer, many years before. Bless her heart, she now has come to terms with it and has accepted it.

kgolds

CHAPTER FIVE

Work

"Working gave me normalcy."

Fun Lover

Some women find that dealing with breast cancer causes them to reorder their priorities, with work getting bumped down a peg or two. Others are compelled to become even more zealous in pursuing their careers. I wish I could say cancer tempered my work drive, but it didn't; what happened was more of an adjustment between work and play, a fine-tuning of the Life Dial. I didn't want my life to be different—I wanted to get on with things, to continue as though little had changed. At the office I was uncomfortable being treated differently because of my breast cancer, and the truth is that I don't think I was given a free pass. My immediate boss was temperamentally neither warm nor very understanding, and I often felt guilty leaving work early because of, say, fatigue from radiation sessions. Fortunately, this was offset by the head of our company, whose every word and action conveyed sympathy and compassion, and so I shared with him some of my most personal feelings while juggling work and illness. In all, I would say that I went out of my way to avoid receiving preferential treatment. Was this wise? Was I being unnecessarily private? Was I denying myself some extra care during a time of extra need? No, yes, *and perhaps. Happily, plenty of colleagues were kind and solicitous and tolerated my occasional lapses. Looking back, work didn't make my days harder, but in truth made them more bearable.*

Thanks in part to the feminism of the 1970s, women and work have become as primary as women and marriage. It's been more than thirty years since Shirley Conran wrote Superwoman, *the first book that codified the woman who wanted it all—a career, marriage and children, time for friendships, time alone. The book is out of print, but the term* superwoman *has as much currency today as it did then. How many women found they were trying to be that "superwoman" at work and in their personal lives when dealing with breast cancer, or that mixing the professional with the personal was like trying to mix oil with water? Was it easy or hard telling a boss or colleague about your illness? How did* you *handle it?*

OH, TO BE NORMAL!

For most of my life, I associated the word normal with boring. That changed once I was diagnosed, and then I longed to be like everybody else my age and be "normal." Weirdly, it took being at the office to feel normal; there I could shut out the worries and fear that swirled around me at home, which had come to symbolize the "sick" me.

> "I was so focused on my job that I didn't have time to dwell on my treatments."
>
> DianaRmn

I must say that all those people I was in contact with at work were incredibly supportive and kind. I forced myself to come to work as often as I possibly could. I needed interaction with people and I needed to be in the midst of some normalcy.

Jacquie

I had accepted a new job before my diagnosis and was scheduled to start three weeks after diagnosis. It was a transfer opportunity and I spoke with my new department about my diagnosis and what I knew for sure, which wasn't much. They took a chance and let me keep the position they had offered me. They were incredibly supportive and I worked very hard to learn my new position. In many ways it was a gift. I was so focused on my job that I didn't have time to dwell on my treatments.

DianaRmn

At my last treatment, everyone in the office applauded! I didn't like the special attention; it's that striving for normalcy, which, of course, it's not. Somehow I just wanted the treatments to be over and if no one paid attention, all the better.

betty

Since I'm an ED I report to a board of directors. When I first got the diagnosis I was going to quit work. I didn't think they should have to deal with someone who couldn't give it her all. I told the chair of the board and he then told the rest of the board members. I had a board meeting shortly thereafter and they were amazing. Very supportive and genuinely caring. All of this support didn't stop. It continued throughout my treatments. I was very lucky and was able to work throughout my chemo treatments. Working gave me normalcy.

It has been a hard year for our organization but never once have any of them complained.

Fun Lover

WORK, THE "PORT IN THE STORM"

Work was my port in the storm. I only told my boss. I requested that people only be informed on a need-to-know basis. The workplace became my refuge. People didn't know so they all treated me with the same admiration or disgust as usual. Work was the only place I felt totally in control, totally in charge. It was such a tame animal compared to the beast that lurked outside the confines of my 9 to 5. Work was my coffee break from chaos.

Delivered

> "Work was my coffee break from chaos."
>
> Delivered

Everyone at work was great. But I felt obligated to come to work even if I didn't feel good because our office is so small and I am the office manager. I think work saved my sanity. I focused on work and not on the fact that I felt so badly.

DollyD

I was able to work, except for chemo days and surgery. I didn't feel my best a lot of the time but I would have felt bad at home too. People kept asking me, why are you working? 1) Money. Bills are still coming in, and more now with the doctor bills; 2) Normal. I wanted things to be as normal as could be; 3) Helped keep my mind off my problems. My doctor really never gave me any restrictions, said to do what I felt like. I guess he knew I would anyway. I got on FMLA [Family Medical Leave Act] at work so the time I was off didn't count against my attendance.

Believer

Believer, you have summed it up so neatly! I can completely understand wanting to take time off to focus on yourself, heal and maybe take care of yourself in ways not possible when working full time, but for me, work has been a good part of my mental salvation. I would have felt worse at home dwelling on my illness than I have done while on the job. My boss has been great to me the past couple of weeks, but then I am here in the office keeping up with everything, even though I have sore feet and a very sore mouth. So we'll take it one day at a time.

songbird

ACTS OF KINDNESS, GIFTS OF GENEROSITY

There are so many ways in which coworkers show thoughtfulness—cards, a gift certificate for dining out, even chipping in with housecleaning and donating their vacation time.

> "A good support team, whether it's family, friends, or coworkers, has everything to do with your healing process."
>
> river

During my chemo, my colleagues used to send cards, e-mails, flowers, and food to help me get through my months of battling this disease. One day, I got an audio tape in the mail—one woman at work went to all the people in our division and in some other divisions and recorded them greeting me and wishing me well. They even sang a song to me.

Jacquie

The first people I told at work were the 2 other women in my department. When I phoned my boss to tell her that it was cancer, she said, "Oh, sh*t!" The next words were "What can we do for you?" She was such an advocate for me. We do not have any provision for donating sick leave to others, and she tried her best to change that policy. When we finally were told that it was illegal in our situation after getting an opinion from the auditor of our state, she took up a collection among coworkers. Between them, they presented me with over $1,000 to help with expenses! That was soooo humbling.

The other thing my coworkers did was to rally and clean my house from top to bottom. A crew of 8 or so women came in one afternoon while I was gone, and vacuumed, mopped, washed windows, dusted, scrubbed bathtubs, and so on. My boss had organized them and then provided dinner for them afterward.

buckeyemom

I went to work and told my manager and asked her not to tell any of my coworkers yet. After talking to my doctor and deciding what was next I then called her to let her know that it was okay to tell the rest of my coworkers. Because we are all so close at work I later found out that they all started crying and that was why I didn't want to be there when they were told. A good support team, whether it's family, friends, or coworkers, has everything to do with your healing process. Whenever people asked me if I was okay, I would tell them no but I will be.

river

My coworkers were and have been very supportive. I took advantage of the Family Leave Act and stayed home a few weeks before surgery and the 8 weeks after surgery. I worked through my chemo and everyone was very cautious of exposing me to any other illnesses. Many people throughout our hospital donated their vacation time to me so that I would keep getting a paycheck while I was out. They also got together and gave a certificate to a local restaurant that I or my family could use whenever I wasn't able to make dinner.

They continue to support me through donations and participating in walks and by allowing me to take time off from the day to go and talk to others about breast cancer. The coworkers that I am closest to even wear pink ribbons on their I.D. badges. I am very grateful to have such support.

koalas

LESSONS LEARNED "ON THE JOB"

I sat with my boss and explained the diagnosis and how I wanted to handle the situation with others. I personally met with direct reports in a group, face-to-face, early in the day and purposefully told them my door was open to them the rest of the day for any additional thoughts or questions (which some did take advantage of). But above all, let there be humor and laughter around the office on my account or for any other good reason!

The rest of my truth is this: before my experience with breast cancer I would probably have been one of those individuals who behaved "badly." I would have feared talking to the person as though I could catch cancer. I was a complete idiot discussing dying and my own death, particularly. Which is why I know I am truly blessed because all of my good, close friends stayed with me, even my coworkers. They behaved "well." I would like to think I helped them though, by setting the tone and then walking my talk. This experience is one of the chief reasons I am now so amazed by life. How is it one who has behaved "badly" could be deserving of such good friends?

Picassa

People say to me that I'm always positive and optimistic. Well, I chose to be that way because that's what it takes to succeed, that's the kind of person people want to be with, and I want people to like me. So there! After being diagnosed with cancer I received a letter from a woman manager in my company who I considered a major competitor (she got a job I wanted) and she wrote, "If anyone can beat this you will because you are the most optimistic person I know." I was flabbergasted.

Noel

THE CANCER CONNECTION

Talk about silver linings! Sometimes even the office can double as both a sister-hood and brotherhood of people who have experienced cancer.

> "It seems most everyone has a family member or friend that has gone through breast cancer treatments."
>
> mtn woman

At work, I first told my boss. I had been working for him for about 10 years when I got the news. I called to tell him and he told me how sorry he was. He had been a great mentor to me in my career, but had always been more about work and kept his personal life and emotions very personal. He was calm and collected and he said, "You can beat this. I am living proof that cancer can be beaten." I had worked for him for 10 years and not known that he had been diagnosed with testicular cancer when he was in his mid-twenties. So we were able to share some of our experiences along the way.

junebug

The company where I have worked for over 20 years is one of my biggest support teams, from my coworkers to my supervisor to my executive VP. I am set up with all my computer privileges at home and can work from here to make up lost time if I feel like it. It gives me the luxury of being able to work for a while and then take a rest if I need to on the days right after chemo. One man who lost his wife to this battle came by to talk and offer support to my husband if he might need to talk to another man about what it was to help someone fighting breast cancer. This same man also told me that breast cancer did not have a clue what an awesome opponent it had chosen when it picked on me.

Scottie

I was fortunate to be working for a large company with great benefits and so taking 3 to 4 weeks off wasn't a problem. Besides, I was working from home as soon as I could get online or on the phone. Telling the rest of the leadership team I worked with was pretty easy and all were supportive and helpful. About 5 years later I was involved with a diversity issues group and it turned out that several of us had breast cancer. Another woman in the group asked four of us if we would share our stories so that others in our company could benefit from our experiences (much like this book) and what came out of that was a most incredible video that received pretty wide use and created strong bonds among the four "stars" of the film.

Susan

IMPORTANCE OF PRIVATE LIFE OVER WORK

The first person I told at work was my boss since I would be needing time off for pre-op testing, etc. Her main concern was how many times I would be out of the office, how long I would be out for my surgery and recovery, and who would handle my work while I was gone. I was very open about my condition and did not feel strange about anyone knowing. (Of course I thought that the Big C days were long in the past!) When I lost my position and became unemployed I thought seriously about changing careers. I have decided to downgrade the position I am looking for to a lower level so I can work more reasonable hours. My private life has become much more important to me than my professional success.

clk913

I never thought of changing careers, only ending one. Because of the memory problems and the possibility of shortened life, I want to take early retirement. I want to have my "golden" years, even if I have to grab them now. That sounds more pessimistic than I am. This disease has just changed my priorities.

ritavv

> "My private life has become much more important to me than my professional success."
>
> clk913

I had to quit my job during treatment due to the debilitating fatigue that I experienced from the chemo and rads. I was unable to physically handle staying in an upright position for more than 2 to 3 hours at a time so therefore I was unable to handle the commute and demands of my job. Truthfully, I was so focused on surviving that I didn't give a rat's behind about working.

Warrior

To me, the cancer was a big wake-up call that said that I'd worked a stressful job long enough and now I should get away from that and be at home closer to my kids.

lily987654

WHEN CHANGING JOBS IS THE RIGHT THING TO DO

I don't want to go back to what I did before—too stressful. What do you say when an employer asks you why you're applying for something that you're "overqualified" for?

kimmytoo

I work at a breast care center. As I spend my days typing about women being diagnosed with breast cancer, their recurrence and their fears of recurrence, I wonder if I need to move on to something different as far as work. Sometimes I feel like it's enough just having it, but to have to hear about it every day, sometimes I feel like screaming. It's educational, but sometimes you can have too much knowledge, ya know? I kind of like to forget that I've had cancer sometimes. I know I'll never actually forget it, but to be reminded every day maybe isn't the best thing for me right now.

Squirrel

Wanting to stop work but not wanting to sacrifice your career

I took a few weeks off following my surgery and have since returned to work part-time during chemo. I have a lot of conflicting feelings about working during treatment. On the other hand, I'm afraid that by not working full time I'll lose ground professionally or not be taken seriously as a "player." And I sometimes feel guilty when I hear about other women who continue to work full time during treatment, like I'm not being a good role model or an "inspiration" because I'm not a superwoman. A job or career change would mean a significant reduction in salary, but I am considering it.

Towanda

I'm very tired after going back to work; it feels good to be back but my arm hurts and swells daily. I just don't know if it's going to let me work at what I do best. I'm a cook and cook for 90 to 120 people and that's a lot of heavy lifting. I just don't want to quit; I think it will make me feel like I'm giving up and I don't want to feel like that. My hubby constantly tells me I'm struggling too much and not to do as much but it's not me to not pull my weight. Some days I hurt so bad I want to give up and other days I just don't know what I'd do if I didn't work . . . . . sigh . . . . . decisions, decisions, decisions.

lilybelle2

BEING KNOWN AROUND THE OFFICE AS A WOMAN WITH BREAST CANCER

I don't want to waste any energy on trying to hide what has happened to me so that others won't feel uncomfortable. It also made me face the notion very publicly that I am vulnerable as we all are to illness and other things beyond our control.

sawiam

I wanted the staff and the students to see that a diagnosis of breast cancer was not necessarily a death sentence. They rejoiced when my hair started to grow back. They commiserated when I was pale and tired from chemo. This spring, one year after my diagnosis, I was the guest speaker for a group of our 4th and 5th graders who were participating in an American Cancer Society fundraising walk/run. They dedicated their fundraising in my honor, which was very touching for me.

I also became the "go-to" person for others who had suspicious mammograms or needed biopsies and for a couple women whose mothers were diagnosed with breast cancer during the same period that I was going through treatment. They knew that I could *really* understand their fears and concerns.

kamaha

I always have felt that it was okay for anyone to know about what I was going through, and I am glad that I decided to handle it that way, as I have had an incredible amount of support from people at work, including people that I hardly knew. It has been one of the best things about this horrible disease.

Grown Mom

Being "the woman with breast cancer" at work felt a little strange as I had always been "the athlete" at work before my diagnosis. I think that was hard for people to square with. But everyone was so great. My biggest concern was that people would treat me differently. I didn't want them to think I couldn't do my job just because I had cancer. In fact, I am in the process of changing careers as a direct result of my diagnosis. I have decided to become an oncology nurse. I realized I want to be a part of the cancer community for the rest of my life.

triathletesurvivor

For a person who never has been able to take naps, I needed one every afternoon. Instead I'd lay my head down on my desk for about 15 minutes and then push on. My management was very understanding. I have no problem with being the woman with breast cancer. I wear my survivorship with pride. I even have a gold chain with a pink ribbon charm on it that I wear sometimes.

ritavv

I don't feel uncomfortable about being known as the person with breast cancer. I think at first they were all waiting to see when I was going to die. It has been three years now and I am stronger than I ever was. This in itself is helpful for those who have to face this disease or have someone in their family face it. I work in a profession where things are by necessity kept under control and cancer, as we all know, cannot be controlled. That is my struggle, every day in big ways and in small, in dealing with this illness. I take one day at a time.

sawiam

Sometimes you have an opportunity to set a good example for others

I am an 11th grade teacher. When I told my principal, I asked him to call a meeting of the faculty so that I could tell them I had been diagnosed with a rare, aggressive cancer called inflammatory breast cancer. I also told each class so they knew the facts. I also told them that I would be glad to answer questions when I returned and they could call me just like before if they needed help. They all accepted it so well. In fact, when I lost my hair, several students asked if I would take my wig off and show them my bald head. I did. It was not always easy, but what was important to me was to help teach the students how to handle adversity when it came your way. By setting a positive example, maybe they would learn that they too could pick themselves up and move on when faced with some of the problems that teenagers face in today's world.

Linda

When "don't ask, don't tell" isn't an option

Saying the words *breast cancer* was so incredibly difficult for me. I was a nervous wreck going to work the first day after my diagnosis. I really just wanted to keep it my own little secret. But I knew that was not possible. I'm in the United States Air Force. There's not much that happens in an active duty person's life that isn't known in the workplace. I work in a predominately male shop. There's little room in our shop for slackers so I knew my secret would have to be known or I would be on the receiving end of a lot of comments for missing work. I decided to tell my flight commander. I told him I needed to speak to him in private. He immediately made time for me. I was an emotional mess during the meeting. I would lose my composure, regain my composure, lose my composure, and regain it again. It was an emotional roller-coaster, like most of my experience so far with breast cancer. My flight commander was amazing. He responded exactly the way I needed. He asked me if I wanted him to keep it private. I told him I wanted the rest of the shop to know but there was no way I could tell them. He volunteered to tell the rest of the group. I was so thankful for that. Everyone at work was supportive. They offered to mow my grass, make dinner, babysit my daughter. You name it, they were willing to help.

D'sMom

Conditional support and acceptance

At the time of my diagnosis, I was working in a small office with just me and the boss. So I told him. He was very good at first. I took a week of sick leave after the lumpectomy. But during that week, I got flowers from the district and regional managers. When I told my boss, he said he knew and he told them "they were making a big deal out of something that wasn't a big deal." I was highly offended. Once the radiation was over, I was supposed to be well and over it and ready to work overtime whenever he chose. I wound up in an awful depression to the point that I started seeing a therapist once a week and my boss objected *strongly* to all my time off. I actually quit the job because of his attitude.

I am now working for his competition. I take it a lot easier than I did working for him. I never work overtime. Never. I am not making as much money but I feel sooooooo much better about my job.

Nett

The first time I was diagnosed in 1989 I was in surgery four days later. On my third day after surgery it all hit me. I was lying in my hospital bed, trying to absorb the cancer diagnosis when my boss (and owner of the company) called to tell me that he had cleaned my desk out. I guess he thought he was being helpful, but I felt like he was telling me he didn't think I was going to make it. It took me an hour to stop crying. I made a vow to leave that job as soon as I could get medical coverage elsewhere, which meant going six months without a doctor's visit. It turned out to be a blessing in disguise. I went back to school and got my teaching certificate and doubled my salary. Lots more fun working with kids.

beachbooks

Mixed bag

When I got to work I told the other 7 people in my office and called the main office to tell the general manager. I am not the kind of person to keep things like that to myself. The response was good and bad. Everyone was very supportive. I was an hourly employee with only a little sick time available but when I had chemo they paid me for the days I was off from that. The bad part was that it was a smoking office. People could smoke at their desks and did. They wouldn't even consider going outside to smoke. So while I appreciated the "support" I couldn't get over the fact that even a coworker's cancer diagnosis was not enough to make them change.

Lisabe

I work as a RN, and for the most part I have a hard time getting time off to go to doctor's appointments etc. It cracks me up I work in healthcare yet they don't support you in maintaining good health.

Alexk48

JOB SECURITY

At my recurrence I was at my present job working as a technical writer, a subject I had taught at our local university. At about 1 year post-recurrence, everyone in my unit except me received a promotion, including a woman who could not spell, let alone put a paragraph together without extensive editing. I asked why I did not get a raise, and my manager said, "It's too bad you got sick." My e-mail to HR resulted in my promotion the next day.

I wonder at times if it was wise to be open, perhaps it would be easier to just be quiet. Then I recall my grandmother who died of breast cancer without telling anyone, and I stand up straight, look people in the eye, and expect fair treatment and dare anyone to pity me.

Toni

PART TWO

Living with Breast Cancer

CHAPTER SIX

Being Womanly

"I behold myself womanly."

Jackjoy

What does it mean to be womanly after you've been diagnosed with breast cancer? How does a mastectomy, for example, change the way you think of yourself—are you still attractive to others, and more important still, how do you regard yourself? At various times over the years, my oldest brother will tell me he thinks I'm a "hottie." "Me?" I reply. "At my age? Are you nuts?" Yet it's his way of saying that despite the surgeries and physical changes, he doesn't think that my attractiveness is in any way diminished. He's a nice guy. Yet I do feel compromised, even though rationally I know this is nonsense. There's a little bit of me in each of the topics addressed in this chapter—I'm annoyed by advertising that defines female beauty according to breast size; I've felt challenged by the changes to my body; and I am adamant that my worth is greater than my parts.

What most "outsiders" don't realize is that a mastectomy isn't just the loss of one or two breasts; oftentimes, the surgery is part of the overall protocol, which might also include radiation, or chemotherapy, and oral medications for years. Then there are the side effects from all

*the treatments and procedures—hair loss, dry skin, joint pain, insuf-
ficient bone density, weight gain, mood changes. In other words, the
changes are ongoing, and so is our assessment of our beauty and self.
How much, we ask ourselves over the course of this journey, do looks
matter?*

*This is one of the richest chapters in the book. Asking a woman
how she feels about being womanly is like asking a child how she feels
about candy—a response is guaranteed. The issues that attach themselves to this topic depend in part on where you are in dealing with
your illness, how old you are, and your own inner strength or personal
demons. Self-image and self-worth become worthy sparring partners in
the ongoing debate about what it means to be womanly. In their comments, the women often discuss the (dis)appearance of their breasts,
and they respond to and challenge cultural notions about female sexuality and beauty. However, despite their various struggles and concerns, they are unanimous that being alive is being womanly.*

THE BIG PICTURE

Being womanly (Wom"an*ly, *adv.* In the manner of a woman; with
the grace, tenderness, or affection of a woman. adj: befitting or char-
acteristic of a woman, especially a mature woman; "womanly virtues
of gentleness and compassion" woman. An adult female person).

This is really hard to define. Everyone has to come to terms with
the hand they have been dealt and I guess womanly is like beauty—it
is in the eyes of the beholder and I behold myself womanly. What it all
boils down to is the only approval that is necessary in this life is yours.

Jackjoy

It disturbs me to see magazines, TV, and other types of ads using
women with large breasts in revealing clothing as the way to enhance
sales of their products. What does this message send to the public?
And for those of us with children, young or old, how does this shape

their value of the female body? I talk with many women with breast cancer, particularly those who have had a mastectomy (single or double), and it really seems to tick them off especially. Women are more than voluptuous breasts.

Being womanly comes from within—I don't feel defined by my breasts, or lack of having breasts. Feeling womanly is a state of mind most of the time, but I do recall feeling more compromised in my opinion in this area in the few years following my diagnosis,* so I guess our concepts evolve over time. Time can be a great healer.

Eileen

*Eileen was only thirty-four at the time she was diagnosed with Stage 2B cancer in 1991.

> "After breast cancer, we are more womanly than ever and we must each listen to our own inner woman and honor her and the wisdom she's found in the suffering from breast cancer."
>
> 2peke

I have been pregnant 4 times, "sort of" thin, and often heavy. I loved to look sexy "before," but have learned to live with my body as it is. What makes me feel womanly is still dressing nicely and how I feel inside!

Mom of 4 Boys

> "What it all boils down to is the only approval that is necessary in this life is yours."
>
> Jackjoy

Being single has made feeling womanly, or sexy, less of an issue than it would if I was still married, or had a boyfriend. I didn't date during my separation, and my divorce was finalized after my diagnosis. I did go on my first date in over 20 years during chemo. In fact, I went on several dates with the same man and had a great time. I felt more like a normal person than I had in months. I was more self-conscious and less self-confident when I was young and thin, with perky, B-cup breasts, than I am now.

kathi1964

> "Being womanly to me is to be feminine without needing to wear frilly things, motherly even if you do not have children of your own but care about others, and being the foundation of my family."
>
> dreamer

For some of us who lived through the 1950s and the era (well, one of them) of hourglass figures, breasts were what defined femininity. We all know menstruation was a "curse," but breasts gave us status. I still remember the first girl in my class who wore a bra, and she flaunted it. The rest of us were envious. I lived for the day when I could look down at my feet and not see them. Then came the liberated days of the late 60s—we threw away our bras and deliberately wore clothes that emphasized the fact.

So now that our most womanly part, that with which we nourish our children (and we could go on about why men love breasts because they never grow up, et cetera), has been desecrated, what do we do? How do we go on?

Myself, I like to indulge in pretty, frilly bras. Yeah, I don't look the same in them, but they make me feel like the physical woman I used to be.

2peke

> "I bet you most definitions of what it is to be
> 'womanly' have been written by men."
>
> reginabu

I don't have a concept of "being womanly." I just am who I am, and I happen to also be a woman. But sometimes I think I'm not a very sexy woman anymore.

kamaha

As far as my concept of "being womanly," I feel that anything a woman wants to do, enjoys doing, feels comfortable doing, is womanly.

KeyWoman

Self-image is an important factor in this disease: we just don't lose a breast, we sometimes lose the image of beauty. It's important if you're in a relationship that your partner tells you that you're beautiful when you're bald, if you had a breast removed, even when you're feeling at your worst. Having someone admire the strength that you have to look and feel beautiful.

Martha Survivor

OUR BODIES, OUR BREASTS

Pro or con, intense or indifferent, every woman who lives with breast cancer has an opinion about her breasts.

> "No doubt about it, I feel way more womanly
> with breasts."
>
> Susana

> "Confidence and self-love is much sexier than a hot body in the long run anyway."
>
> MCN

Susana and Agent99: two sides of the same coin

I feel totally mutilated as a woman after bilateral mastectomies. What I have on the front of me, done by a pair of top national plastic surgeons, are "two grapefruit halves on a washboard." Fixed, hard, numb, tight, and nippleless. Aren't breasts supposed to be soft, warm, jiggly, bouncy, and pointy? My physicians assured me that I would be left with "breasts as good as or better than before, even a bit more adolescent." Well, excuse me, but they were dead wrong. And now I am afraid to have the whole thing redone because frankly I doubt that anyone could truly make it better.

My breasts have been amputated to save my life, a sacrifice I was willing to make and would make again. But no doubt about it, the loss continues to be horrendous. Do I feel womanly? Well, yes, in some ways, but NO! NO! NO! in the most glorious basic breast-y Venus de Milo way. Not only can I not feed babies, but I can't even offer them a soft, warm bosom to cuddle or cry into. When the doctor said I would lose some sensation, I didn't know he meant that I would be completely numb across my whole chest forever, never again able to feel the touch of a lover, the closeness of a hug or slow dance, not even cold water or pain.

Of course it is possible to create a new self-image which includes all the depth and even richness of the cancer experience, along with the wounds, and I have done that. I am rock solid, healthy, and happy enough. But would I love to have my breasts back? *Yes!! Yes!!* And . . . . ooh . . . aah . . . how sweetly I would cherish them this time! No doubt about it, I feel way more womanly with breasts.

Susana

I feel like taking off my shirt and showing people my one breast and saying, *this* is what breast cancer looks like. There's nothing pretty about it. Of course any man worth anything will still love us for who we are, but it is simply unnatural to go around with one breast. I'm sure I'll adapt, and I am planning on having reconstruction. But I miss my beautiful healthy breast, soft, perfect, used to feed my baby and to give me pleasure. I was butchered (and mind you, my result is cosmetically really quite good), this treatment is barbaric, and I will *not* sit quietly and say I'm just grateful to be alive. I'll be grateful when the solution to the disease isn't to chop off a body part and then systemically poison and burn women.

Agent99

"Our breasts are a part of our body, but even if I looked like a man, what is inside of me makes me a woman."

jester

These women are all under the age of forty

It bears repeating that as awful as breast cancer is for any woman, a woman's sense of her natural beauty is considerably impacted when she's not even yet forty.

I know what the "right" or "healthy" answers are to fill in here but that would not be honest. Before my diagnosis, I loved my breasts. Firm, symmetrical 34Ds. I was confident in a V-neck top and wore close-fitting shirts.

Then my breast betrayed me. I had recently stopped nursing my daughter when I discovered a 3.7 cm tumor while showering. I chose not to have a lumpectomy because the plastic surgeon said I would be disfigured and have few options to improve the outcome. So I chose the tram (my surgeon said it would provide the most "natural look-ing" outcome). I am one of that small percentage of people who had many complications—severe necrosis that required three more sur-geries with skin grafts. Just last week, I got an implant. My new breast does not look like the other one nor is it as good as the original. I do not have the option of nipple reconstruction because of the grafts. I now wear loose-fitting clothing and have resigned myself to never having sex again. I am not sure if this outcome is truly better than the lumpectomy would have been or not.

I don't know about feeling less womanly but I definitely feel more like 60 than my actual 32 years. I work in an office where 90 percent of the employees are under 35. Just having cancer was shocking enough without all of the close stares at my chest, as much from women as from men.

jennie

My image of myself has changed enormously since I lost both my breasts at 36. I am 5' 9", 145 lbs., Canadian, with an amazing hus-band and 2 children. When I look in the mirror and see no breasts (I was a 36C), it all still seems rather surreal. No reconstruction feels right for me at this time. But of course, I cannot deny I miss my breasts greatly. When I look at the big picture, *life* and *health* are what's most important, the rest is all secondary. But that is not to say that I still feel inadequate at times, particularly when I see movies with love scenes of women's beautiful perfect breasts being caressed by their lovers, that's very difficult for me, that's when I have a meltdown be-cause my heart aches for my breasts again. So I'm careful what I watch on TV.

Big Red

I was all hair and tits in my 20s and early 30s and now my mane is gone and the breasts I waited for all through high school that showed up abundantly and beautifully are flaccid and scarred, these once-beautiful mounds that my friends would chide me for peeking at every so often, or caressing; these breasts that paid for my schooling (okay, I never said I made the wisest decisions concerning them) and gave me the financial freedom to be able to nurse my mother to her death by lung cancer, I won't even touch, not even for a self-breast exam. I am petrified I will feel something and the nightmare will begin again.

Is it better to mourn something you had or didn't have? Who can say? I have had people ask me if I think my cancer is God's punishment for the way I conducted myself when younger. The thought crossed my mind, but jeez, get real—the prisons are full of cancer-free pedophiles, rapists, and murderers.

Mamaper

Body image and society

A few years ago I found a card in a bookstore with a picture of a woman who had had a double mastectomy, arms over her head, a joyful posture, and terrific statement. I championed her! But I can't do that.

Al

> "It disturbs me to see magazines, TV, and other types of ads using women with large breasts in revealing clothing as the way to enhance sales of their products."
>
> Eileen

I don't think I want to be a fantasy model as much as I want to look like a normal healthy woman, because that is how I want to see myself. After a bilateral mastectomy, my chest isn't just flat, it's concave.

This is why I am choosing reconstruction. It's for me, not "society." I want to be as whole as I can.

tootie

Why is it so difficult to function in our society with only one (or no) breast(s)? I worry about the reaction of others. Am I the only one who struggles with the public side of this?

cj

I struggle with this issue as well. Even though my boobs were not that large, some clothes, especially dresses, just do not hang right without a bra and prosthesis or something stuffed in the bra. Also, I look odd in a bathing suit unless it has stiff cups. I study preadolescent girls and wonder why they look great boobless, maybe because they don't have curves other places. I don't know. In the locker room at the Y where I swim, most women walk around naked. I don't because I don't want to frighten anyone. I am happy with the way I look, but it could be scary to someone who has not been through what we have been through.

Kay

CJ,

I think you should worry about what *you* are comfortable with, and to hell with what others think. I have one breast. I don't wear a prosthesis. People can accept me for *me* or not, it's their choice. I am not going to go out of my way, have another surgery, with the hopes someone may accept me based on having two breasts. The people that know me accept my feelings, although they may not agree. The people that I meet rarely notice I have only one breast. If they do notice and have the guts to ask, I tell them I had breast cancer and a mastectomy, and that's the end of it.

Best,

KeyWoman

Positive outlook — beauty from within

For these women, the glass is half-full, not half-empty. They are proactive, frank, and determined.

Believe it or not (and I know some will think I was crazy), but once all of my treatments were complete and my surgeries were done I went in for one more and that was to get another implant in my good breast. I figured that if I was going to go through all this *crap*, I might as well go for the gold.

    Krista

> "Cancer is something I can live with and even though I would not wish it on anyone, in my case I think it has made me a stronger, more self-confident person."
>
>   Marybe

Yes, one of my breasts has a dimple and is still blue from the sentinel node biopsy but it's unique. Not another one like it out there.

    Sara C

> "I believe breast cancer was the final piece of the puzzle I needed to see that I am a beautiful woman no matter what the outside looks like."
>
>   Lisabe

I remind myself and all who will listen that my daddy died at age 34 from brain cancer. You can take a breast off; you can't take a brain out.

    Mawsquaw

> "It is ironic that something which left me so disfigured on the outside has left me so whole on the inside."
>
> ARSteach

I don't feel sexy nor do I want to. This has changed the way I see myself in all areas of my life. I am smart, strong, caring, determined, and that is all that matters to me now. What makes me feel good is being with my family and not taking the little things for granted. It seemed to me that this spring the grass was greener and the flowers were brighter and the sky was bluer.

DollyD

I don't mean to sound like a Pollyanna about this but for me losing a breast wasn't all that big a deal. My mother had a radical mastectomy with complete chest wall removal and all I was facing was a modified radical—just didn't compare on the same scale to her disfigurement. It wasn't like I needed the breast in the same way I needed other body parts so I was pretty grateful to lose something I really could do without.

There is no doubt I've had a spiritual renewal, strengthened relationships, learned to slow down just a teensy bit, and now have this new kinship with others facing breast cancer that allows me to share the same kind of support that I came to know during my cancer. I do consider those blessings, and to join in this "group hug."

Susan

Courage

I am a woman of enormous strength and courage. I am a woman who happens to be a wife, mother, and daughter who has breast cancer. I really never cared what other people thought about how I looked before I had breast cancer, and now I really don't care how anyone else thinks I look. Does that mean that I don't get upset about seeing the scars, or angry when I would really like to wear a strapless dress and can't? No, of course I do. However, I refuse to dwell on that kind of superficial nonsense. I am alive, and that's all that matters to me.

Warrior

> "I can add courage to my resume."
>
> Gram K

I get to be a hero to myself for never giving up. We don't always get to be heroes to ourselves. It is very spiritual. I also get to add to the legacy I leave to my children, grandchildren, friends, and family.

Greatful2b

Breast cancer has changed my physical appearance, but that's not who I am. I am proud that I can add courage to my resume. It's not easy to stay positive through treatment, but I did it. It's not easy to be the only one in the room wearing a hat or baseball cap and still have a smile on your face, and it's not easy being in a room full of people and being the only one asked "So, how are you doing?" I know I am stronger because of the last three years. You never know how much you can handle until you have to.

Gram K

BETTER THAN BEFORE

Remarkably, some women describe becoming better human beings due to having breast cancer. This is not about seeking the proverbial silver lining, but about doing real work to improve their lives.

> "I do feel like a woman again: strong, sexy, smart, wanted, attractive, and full of life."
> jonessugar

In some ways, my life didn't really begin until I had breast cancer. Yes, the fears, pain, disfiguration, and sense of loss were huge, but when I emerged on the other side of treatment, I was strong, fully alive, and my self-worth was at its highest. I have also learned to protect my boundaries from other people. I am no longer willing to let toxic people impose upon me. I fought too hard for this life to give up any aspect of it to those who don't treat me with love and respect. I may never be innocent again, but I will also never be weak again.

happytobehere

Because of my relationship starting soon after surgery with my current boyfriend and him not even flinching when he first saw my body (boob and tummy incision), body image has not been a big deal for me. In fact, I am probably more comfortable in my body than before surgery because I have chosen to look at it unlike ever before.

On the whole I feel great about my body now. Better than before, in part due to my participating in an exercise program. I may well be more fit now than ever before. Besides, I figure there is not much I can do about it now, so I just work to accept what is.

Picassa

MY PARTS ARE NOT THE SUM OF ME . . .

Imagine you are holding an apple. You peel that apple—without the skin, is it still an apple? You then cut it into quarters—is it still an apple? And finally, you eat half the apple. Has the character, the essence of that apple, disappeared?

"I was a babe before my surgeries. I'm a babe now. Attitude is everything."

MoxieAir

"I can't erase the scars, but I can enhance the other parts of myself."

reginabu

A woman is all the things that are inside her. She has a mind that she has used to gain knowledge. She has knowledge that she has used to show her talents, whatever they may be. And most important of all, she has heart. Our sexuality is not centered in our breasts. Uh-oh, I will get off the soap box.

NMRose

"Cancer surgery has changed me physically, but that is not who I am."

Susie

"I am not my breast"

"I am not my breast." I said that on Day 1, and I haven't wavered one bit. I have a small frame and I get away without even wearing a prosthesis. My blouses have two pockets. If I have an important event, or want pointy breasts, I'll concede to wearing a bra with a prosthesis. Otherwise, I am comfortable in dress, manner, attitude, and self-image.

If anything, I feel more womanly because I don't care about the little things. What is important to enjoying a happy and full life has nothing to do with boobs, wrinkles, even youth. One thing this disease does for you is to help get your priorities straight. The concept of being womanly, of self-worth, should all be in your heart and mind.

mimi

Mimi,

I just love your "I am not my breast" statement. It is both inspirational and hilarious; thinking of myself as nothing more than a mound of breast tissue (conjures up images of the old movie *The Blob*) made me laugh out loud. The coping techniques you mention like pockets on blouses are ones I've used and each time I come up with something or steal shamelessly from someone else's good idea it feels like a victory of sorts. I figure there is no such thing as a perfect body anyway so I'm not concerned with the way mine now looks. I'm a bit of a fitness nut and have always thought my upper arms looked better than my breasts anyway and it's socially acceptable to show them off in public!! My wonderful partner of 25 years continues to find me physically, mentally, emotionally and spiritually appealing. My essence is unchanged and my self-worth comes from so much more than the size and shape of my breasts.

Who I am is better defined by the way I fill my roles as partner, daughter, aunt, friend, colleague, supporter, caregiver, mentor and more.

Susan

I am a one-man woman, but if I weren't, having no breasts would not stop me if I wanted that kind of relationship. If boobs are all a man is looking at, then find another man because they don't make the woman. Just as the size of a man's—I'll be nice—*manhood* does not make him more of a man than someone else. I believe women are more than a pair of boobs. I will say no more.

NMRose

If all that is important are my breasts and what they look like or if I have them, then the person who thinks that way isn't worth my time or love. I am not my breast, and I am not cancer; they are only pieces of who I am, and small pieces at that. What is my heart like, am I kind, strong, loving, compassionate . . . those are the things that count. That and the fact that I am *alive* and cancer free!!!

    Autumn

Amen to that, Autumn!!!! Our hearts are who we are and you don't have to look very deep to find mine—my hubby says I wear it on my sleeve!!!

    lilybelle2

I always feel sexy when I use my brain.

    JoAnn

I do not see my breasts, my ovaries, or my uterus as what makes me womanly. I am a woman because of the way I think and act.

    Kellyk01

SORTING OUT SELF-WORTH AND SELF-IMAGE

Patting your head and rubbing your belly is a no-brainer compared to sorting out issues of self-image and self-worth. Both are in constant flux, interdependent, and a juggling act of feelings.

> "I am more than scars, or wrinkles. I am heart, I am soul, I feel and love and I hurt and cry and I am only human."
>
>   Princess86

For me self-image (body image) has never been the same as self-worth. I would be awfully depressed if that were the case! Instead my self-worth is wrapped up more into my intellectual accomplishments. That isn't good either because one gets into the mode of feeling they need to accomplish something to be loveable. I guess I've never been your traditional woman; not part of my self-image. So my diagnosis had no impact in that area.

ritavv

I believe breast cancer was the final piece of the puzzle I needed to see that I am a beautiful woman no matter what the outside looks like. When I was younger my self-image and self-worth were the same. They were both bad. Today, many years later, because I had breast cancer, my self-image and self-worth are the same again. This time that is great.

Lisabe

> "Whatever problems I had with self-image and self-esteem before the diagnosis—guess what? They are still here afterward."
>
> biblio

I never had much self-worth until I had my son. That is one reason why I wanted more. I always wanted to be a mother, and when I became one, it all fell into place. It was/is the one thing that completes me and makes me the happiest. I have learned through this experience that if nothing else, my life is of value to me and my son, and hopefully to my husband. Anyone else who doesn't feel the same way can just stay away. I no longer feel like I have to put up with others' crap.

Helen

Marybe and Peony compare who they were as teenagers to themselves today

I was never much of a joiner in school and would not do a lot of things because I did not want to try anything I didn't already know how to do for fear I would not be good at it. My mother was always my worst critic in spite of the fact that I know she was also my biggest fan—she somehow managed to do a number on me. Things she used to find wrong with herself, I find have transferred over to me: I complain about my large arms and big thighs just as she did and I won't wear clothes that are too revealing in spite of the fact I have always been told that I have a "cute" shape. Cute is not something I want to be, however I think you just sort of get stuck with that label when you are short.

Since I have never really been happy with my looks, losing a breast did not do much to enhance my self-image. I know there is a lot more involved here than just physical image, but for me it's always been a big part of how I felt about myself. Everyone thinks I have a great personality, am funny, witty, generous, someone people like to be around, but I still remember school days when I did not fit in.

However, I think breast cancer has made me a better person in that I now know physical attributes are not all that important. I have found that people actually think I am an inspiration because of the way I have dealt with my cancer.

To look at me, no one would ever guess that I am Stage IV and it has been 6 years now. Making a difference in others' lives has made a huge difference in mine. Cancer is something I can live with and even though I would not wish it on anyone, in my case I think it has made me a stronger, more self-confident person.

Marybe

Isn't it interesting how a person's perspective changes. When I was in junior high, I would not even go to the mailbox without washing my hair. I have since walked around bald, boobless (no prosthesis), and with multicolored wigs. I think your attitude affects how people see you. I was also teased in school, but now I don't care.

Peony

Self-worth as experienced by goldfinch, DollyD, and metsfan

My self-worth is not a changing thing. I am still a worthy person, with tons of things to contribute to the world. I feel up to the challenge. As an old friend once said to me after her daughter disappeared forever, "These things happen to those of us who can handle it." We just handle it. Even as I see myself conked out on the couch, I still know it's part of handling it. Self-worth is believing in myself. Trusting on all that good stuff from before—upbringing, love, spirit, creative energy, connections, being a positive part of the macrocosm. My self-image is a small part of that bigness.

goldfinch

Self-worth to me is being a productive member of society. I have a good job and I feel that I do it well. I am a good mother and grandmother. I am a good wife and a good daughter. Just because I have cancer doesn't mean that I have no worth now. Do I sound conceited? Sorry if I do, but I get a little defensive about this subject.

DollyD

DollyD,

Conceited? Hardly! Inspiring is more like it. As someone in my support group said yesterday, the idiots on *Survivor* don't have the first clue what the word means. Eating bugs for a million dollars ain't it! Facing a life-threatening condition and refusing to give in is what real surviving is all about.

metsfan

To me self-image and self-worth are not the same. I think I have to separate them to keep me grounded. Who I am physically, even though it has a major impact on my life, is *not* who I am inside. Self-image to me is the outside, the physical, the body, and how I feel about myself as a woman. Self-worth is the inside—the mom, the wife, the daughter—all I have tried to achieve and all I have worked so hard to accomplish. I base my self-worth on the fact that maybe someday somewhere someone is a better person because they met me.

    Princess86

Self-image. Let's see: I can't compete with the girls at the girly bar (never could) and with two mastectomies and tram flap reconstruction and a few added pounds and pain I don't think I ever will. Image is gone and worth I'm working on!

    Mel

My self-image changed drastically when I was doing chemo. And I think my self-worth plummeted at the same time. I felt this way because I was not sure if I was going to die or not. I was still the same person inside, still had the same likes and dislikes, still had the same desires, but the uncertainty unraveled me. Most people my age take their health for granted. I felt like I lost that.

    MJ

MJ was around forty when diagnosed.

I was 25 when I was diagnosed and had only been married for 2 years. It was really hard for me to realize that I was not going to be the youthful 25-year-old anymore. I had to age quickly both emotionally and physically. Where before I had no scars, no skin problems, no fat, I have turned into a scarred, frumpy 28-year-old. My husband doesn't seem to notice my scars anymore, but there is no way he likes them. Not very many other under-30s are having to deal with this.

    My self-worth has grown leaps and bounds. I developed a really strong relationship with God and I know that he has a plan for my life. I really felt like I was given an opportunity to make my life the best it can be and since I can get through breast cancer, I can get through anything!

    jester

A WORK IN PROGRESS:
"MAGGIE THE CAT IS ALIVE. I'M ALIVE!"

In Cat on a Hot Tin Roof, *the young married couple played by Elizabeth Taylor and Paul Newman struggle to achieve happiness. At one point, Newman says to Elizabeth Taylor, "What is the victory of a cat on a hot tin roof?" to which she replies, "Just staying on it, I guess, long as she can."*

> "I played with Barbie dolls as a kid, and part of me always felt like I didn't measure up."
>
> biblio

I am woman. I am sexy. I am boobless. I am pretty. I look a little sick. I am proud. I am scarred. I am good. I am afraid. I am warm. I am still alive. I have bad feelings. I am smart. I know real pain. I am artistic. I deal with lymphedema. I have good feelings. I have blue eyes. I have cancer. I am still alive. *You hear me out there? I am alive.*

biblio

JodieR

> "What makes me feel good about myself? Shopping until I drop! What makes me feel bad? Doctors appointments."
>
> Blessed

Well, this will be tough, but honestly I always felt and saw myself as pretty. I am 6 feet tall and was always told I should be a model. Now comes breast cancer with a modified radical mastectomy. I chose not to do reconstruction. I just did not want to go through anything more than that surgery. I'm a RN and "know too much" about the cons of reconstruction. This said, every day I look at my chest wall and am not particularly pleased with how it looks. With clothes off,

I don't feel pretty. My husband, who was wonderful through all this, is kind enough to say it doesn't bother him, he doesn't mind, it doesn't matter, etc. Now add the 50 pounds that I have gained post-treatment, menopause, and Femera. It is hard, and I feel "silly," vain, and immature to even mention it. "Aren't you just glad to be alive?" Yes, but I would still like to feel like me. I'm working on it. But it's hard.

LynneM

I remember after my surgery different people "came out" to me, told me they had had mastectomies too. My great-aunt told me that prostheses were really annoying and that implants are much more convenient—that made me feel better. But I was so shocked because I wouldn't have known if they hadn't told me. Why don't we get to wear medals, *something* that symbolizes our battles? A breast is not only a body part, it is a gender symbol. So when you lose it, you lose a cultural marker of some sort. You lose a piece of your identity. But if you survive, you pick up the pieces and move on.

biblio

BECOMING INFERTILE

I declined reconstruction of the right breast and never filled the prosthesis prescription. No one can really tell the imbalance. Actually the Lupron putting me into premature menopause at 36 bothered me more than the mastectomy. It is nice not having a period every month, but having bone thinning is not good. I should exercise and be more proactive, but I thought I would not live long enough for it to be an issue. Now I am still here. It hurts me to see people with families and children, knowing I can never have children. After the shock of the floor falling out from under me, I have learned to live with the new course I got enrolled into.

Indeterminate

You know how everybody always thinks they look worse than they actually do? Well, I always thought I looked *better* than I actually did! I think that positive self-image really helped get me through the treatment phase. I went bald and flat-chested the entire time, with no apologies to anybody. (My husband is also bald, and with our matching round faces and overweight bodies, we looked like a couple of salt and pepper shakers trying to make a political statement. We walked by one woman who said, sotto voce to her companion, "Now there go a couple of artists!")

So I don't think my self-image had a lot to do with my self-worth, *but* I have discovered that my fertility did. When I found out I was infertile, I was surprised to find that my self-worth went right out the window. At the bottom of it all, I now honestly feel that there's no point in living. (I know, I know, I'm getting counseling to sort it out.) And, interestingly, that loss of self-worth has destroyed my self-image. When I look in the mirror now, I see all the fat and flaws that I used to overlook. I didn't mean for it to come out this way, but in telling this story, I'm realizing that I'm a walking example of the "beauty doesn't give you self-worth, but self-worth makes you beautiful" theory.

alleeum

THE CHANGE IS A CHALLENGE—BEFORE AND AFTER

Self-image is self-image. I don't have a problem with self-worth. My image is shot. I'm not used to looking this way. My skin color is off, my body is not what it should be. My nails are falling off and my hair is taking forever to grow back. I just want the old me back. Is that crazy or am I crazy? It's like an alien entered this body and shifted it around. Everyone says that I am being hard on myself, that I look okay. But I see something different. I don't see me.

lily

"I miss the old me."

KarenFL

I don't feel as attractive now that I'm bald and have no eyebrows or eyelashes. I know this is just a temporary feeling, though. I find myself wanting to carry around a "before cancer" picture of myself. I want to wear one around my neck. I want to show the young male radiation tech my picture and say, "See, this is the real me." I want to show anyone who does a double take after looking at me.

tinydancer

"I hope someday my mind will accept what I have become since my mastectomy."

finkybinder

Yes, my image of myself changed. I was a 50-year-old who felt like 25 before the cancer and now I am 52 and feel like 70.

Linda

"I do think that regaining self-image and feelings of sexual attractiveness area gradual process—there's a loosening of the ropes."

Toni

Cancer has made me look at myself as I have never done before and I don't really like what I am finding out about myself. I don't have a good self-image. I hate the way I look and will go to great lengths to avoid looking in the mirror. I no longer undress in front of my husband because I feel so ugly. I wear very large sloppy clothes that I hide behind. Maybe someday this will change but I don't really think it will be anytime soon.

kimbasa

> "I just want the old me back. Is that crazy or am I crazy? It's like an alien entered this body and shifted it around."
>
> lily

I have always been a large woman, but have always been very attractive regardless of my size. I didn't like being a large woman, but I really can't remember anything else. I was strong all the way through the treatments, and after the treatments were over, I fell apart. I am learning how to cope so that once again I may be the beautiful woman I was. The image of my womanliness and sexuality has changed. I am learning to mourn the loss and to accept and push forward building a new positive self-image.

Linda

My self-image has not been good since I had my mastectomy in 1979. I get very angry when I try to go shopping for clothes and find everything low cut or sleeveless. I had 2 children get married in the past 2 years and had a terrible time finding a dress that was appropriate for the wedding. It seems that being feminine is based on cleavage in this country. I still look for nightwear that is not revealing and comes up high in the neck. You would think that after 25 years I would have adjusted to this but for some reason I still have problems. I am now just getting so I can exercise without a bra on if I am in my own home. Some things are just hard to accept.

Joyce

My original cancer and my surgery/chemo/radiation were 8 years ago. I did not feel sexually unattractive, but rather sexually uninterested, and I didn't much care what my husband thought of it. I was tired from treatment. Tired from working, parenting, maintaining family life and friendships while in treatment. Tired of an unbalanced body.

Once I grew hair, learned to look at my scars as just a part of me (just as my big feet are a part of me), regained my balance, rested, and engaged in life again, sexual interest returned. I do think that regaining self-image and feelings of sexual attractiveness are a gradual process—there's a loosening of the ropes.

Toni

REDEFINING WHO YOU ARE

"Who am I?" is one of those questions we ask ourselves over the course of our lives. For so many of us, a breast cancer diagnosis brings the identity question into sharp focus—regardless of how hard it is to find an answer.

> "Cancer cannot take away our identity even if it can change the way we look and feel."
>
> songbird

For me self-image is like the gift wrap of the present that is my self-worth. I am more than the breast cancer. I do not define myself by the disease just as I would not want to be defined by my wrap.

Greatful2b

How do you identify yourself? I used to think or say: I'm a teacher, wife, union activist, sister of a person with a disability—those labels that defined who I was—and then I would add attributes that described me, such as articulate, intelligent, competent, organized.

Now I think or say: I'm a breast cancer survivor, retired teacher, wife, etc. Being a breast cancer survivor has become a major part of who I am—it has influenced my actions and my attitudes. I see myself as a cancer survivor and now that's part of how I define who I am.

kamaha

I think my self-worth has skyrocketed since my diagnosis. I have gotten really involved with my kids' school and I can't tell you how good it feels to have my kids want me to work in their classroom or to walk into that school and have 10 little kids come over and give me a hug. Knowing that I have influenced these kids' lives gives me more self-worth than I'd ever imagined. I know that if I should die tomorrow that my legacy will live on through my children, and the children I've had the honor of working with.

DawnMarie

I Am Not My Breast Cancer: Breast Cancer Labels

Once a woman has been diagnosed with breast cancer, matters of identity are reconsidered, revised, and challenged. For some, this is a label akin to a hair shirt, whereas others consider it their personal badge of courage. And is this woman a survivor? Is her experience a "journey," an "adventure," or is it, as one woman writes, "a life I did not anticipate living and one I did not plan"? As for the pink ribbon symbol—the women have plenty to say about that!

For people at my local Y who do not know I had breast cancer, I don't want to be labeled as the "poor girl who had breast cancer twice." Instead, I am just another lap swimmer and I like that.

Kay

"I too detest labels and balk at the term survivor; I feel like a reality program."

–DianaRmn

"I despise labels in any form as they place limitations on who we are as people. You and I had, have, or might have cancer. End of story."

–Hummingbird

"I dislike the survivor label because I think of the women who have not survived. What does that make them—failures?"

–Kellyk01

I think that the hardest blow to my self-image is that people stopped treating me as anything *but* cancer once I was diagnosed. Sometimes I feel that if one more person asks me how I am feeling I will run down the road screaming.

AuburnLiz

"The world needs to put its reaction to breast cancer in perspective and stop regarding those of us with breast cancer as if we were ticking time bombs."

—mountainmomma

WHAT DOES *BREAST CANCER SURVIVOR* MEAN? AND WHAT ABOUT THE WOMEN WHO DIE?

Has anyone else been frustrated by the fact that we are called *survivors*? I don't really know what I did any different than the person who lost her life to cancer. Why am I chosen to live and the person who sits beside me in support group chosen to die?

I am tired of the survivor recognition ceremonies and celebrations for survivors. Did I do something heroic that those who have fought and lost did not do? I am not special because I got breast cancer. My family and friends who put up with my crap when I was diagnosed are my heroes. I want to celebrate that they survived. My marriage survived. They should wear T-shirts that say "Survived the July 2001 Breast Cancer Diagnosis."

jester

I'm not so sure that surviving breast cancer made me a stronger person but having gone through it surely did.

Joanne

Yes, in the beginning when I was first diagnosed, I thought the term *survivor* was absurd. Survivor? Who says I may survive this? And what about those wonderful women who do not survive? They fought just as much as me and they went through so much more. If I do not beat my breast cancer, am I no longer a survivor?

To this day, these questions still remain with me. I now have Stage IV and I have known of 6 women to pass away this year alone. They deserve a much more appropriate word for their fight, their endurance through it all, their bravery. I have many words in my mind that suit them, but they are not wrapped around a pink ribbon all of the time like a *survivor* is. It is not a victory; it is something not celebrated. My heart aches for them and for me.

doowop

I think we are stuck with terms that are used every day to describe us. If we live, we are described as cancer survivors; if we die we are cancer victims.

kathynye

We are survivors not because we beat our battle with cancer but for what we have endured to get where we are today. I lost the love of my life of 4 years. My then 15-year-old daughter was raped by a 30-year-old, my then 18-year-old son went to jail for being young and stupid, and my employer attempted to fire me and I was with a zero income and no insurance for a month. Out of 5 brothers and sisters they all chose to ignore me except for one. My family lives 150 miles away from me so I had little emotional support. I attempted suicide 3 times and the only reason I didn't end up in a mental hospital is because I didn't have insurance. But I *survived*!!! Ladies, that is what I think about when I am called a survivor.

justadame

WHEN IT COMES TO "PRETTY IN PINK," REACTIONS ARE MIXED

In my experience, everyone likes the pink ribbons. It turns breast cancer into something pretty and for those who have been lucky (since we all fight equally hard and want to live, I use the word *lucky*) to survive this disease, it symbolizes something victorious. For me, I just think that if it gets people to spend money for a cure, then bring it on. I support it and my family, friends, and I will always wear them. But I know that breast cancer is more than just a pretty pink ribbon.

doowop

"I'm tired of the whole pink ribbon thing. Make the damned ribbons black."

–Agent99

"I know that breast cancer is more than just a pretty pink ribbon."

–doowop

I'm so glad you guys brought this up! I always thought I was the only one who wasn't on the big pink bandwagon. The pink ribbons used to drive me batty. I got back out into the world in October, and those things were everywhere! Each time I saw one, it was like a punch in the stomach.

That said, we all want awareness and support, and that means we have to put these things out there for the general public to notice. Breast cancer used to be embarrassing; now walks and events and lots of ribbons everywhere make it easier for all of us to tell our stories, get support at work, and comfort our friends and family with knowledge and hope.

So while I refuse to wear that pink-ribbon clothing, etc., because I want to feel so much more than that, I truly appreciate the non-breast cancer survivors/victims/patients who do.

alleeum

Sometimes I feel that there's enormous pressure to be a "good" breast cancer woman and what that means now seems to be *upbeat! positive! glad to be here!* Well, you know what? Of course I'm glad to be here but that doesn't mean my body and soul weren't just raped by treatment.

I'm tired of the whole pink ribbon thing. Make the damned ribbons black.

> Agent99

AND HERE'S A WOMAN WHO TAKES ON THE LABEL OF BREAST CANCER IN ITS MOST GENERIC FORM . . .

Breast cancer is *not* a death sentence!

> artistic person

BREAST CANCER DEBATE 101:
LOOKS DO MATTER VS. DO LOOKS MATTER?

The women consider how they're perceived by the public and also how they see themselves. As to the tired perception that if you look good then you must be fine—bah, humbug, according to some women.

"Mainly, there is very little support for reconstruction. I know it is 'cosmetic' in the strictest sense, but so is wearing clothes and having your hair cut in a becoming style."

A1

"I don't think I fit the mold of what sexy means in our society anymore."

Tracy43

"Beautiful takes many forms!"

Lizzi

"It isn't my desire to upset anyone but I do have that 'this is what breast cancer looks like' mentality."

Agent99

I like to think of myself as a masterpiece in the works. I see my body (which has transformed itself) as a Renaissance woman in a painting. Heck, those bodies are not of what we think the perfect body is today. I had to work hard to see this in myself. I am what I am and if people don't like what they see then they shouldn't look. I know I'm worth so much more than my physical self. My hair and body are only a small part of me. I like to go deeper and think this is only a costume we get for the ball we attend here on earth. Some of us have to shed the costume little by little. Well, my womanhood has remained intact and has actually gotten stronger because of it.

sibling rivalry

Good-bye "sexy," hello "me"

My self-image about how sexy I am has changed. Before having both breasts removed, I spent more time on my looks, clothes, makeup, and being "sexy" for my boyfriend. My figure was society's idea of "sexy" and I worked it! It was fun! I was 39.

After my surgery, I chose not to have any reconstruction and I do not wear a prosthesis. I knew that I would be happier this way. I go flat-chested and don't particularly try to hide the fact. I find that I wear T-shirts and knit tops because they fit better because they don't have darts. So it's very apparent that I have no breasts. Now at 43 with no chest, extra weight, cellulite, and one arm bigger than the other, I don't think I fit the mold of what sexy means in our society anymore.

People say that you shouldn't allow society to dictate what sexy is, but everyone knows that it does so more than any of us want to admit. But my happiness is not dependent on being sexy. Even though "sexy" was fun while it lasted! Feeling less sexy has not changed the fact that I am a huggy-touchy-kissy person. I've always been this way and this never changed.

Although part of my self-image has changed due to having both breasts removed, I don't feel it has changed for the worse. It's just a different self-image now because I'm different now.

Tracy43

At the moment, I am bald, have about 10 eyebrow hairs, zero eyelashes, and one breast. Not a pretty picture. Fortunately, I know there is a lot more to me than what that picture presents and people love me for who I am. I never was much for fussing with my appearance, but I sure used to have great hair and a nice body. I feel even better about my self-worth, knowing I can get through this and the great support I am getting from family and friends.

I think the image part is a little harder on my kids. My nine-year-old often requests that I "wear my hair (wig)" when we go out. I'm hoping I can turn this into a little life lesson about appearances without his being embarrassed of his mom.

Michele

We are truly a society based on looks: if a person looks good then people assume that person is great. Sad, really, but true.

Princess86

That is so true! Everyone bases your health on your looks. I hear that you-look-great shit all of the time. Funny, that is society. I am just very proud to watch my daughter be so caring of others and never base any of her opinions on the way someone looks. I know sometimes when I looked and felt bad during treatment people would talk to me like I was going to die right there in front of them. I would always laugh at that, and those same people now are like, *Oh my God,* you look so *great.* You want to say, "Yeah you thought I would be dead by now." Most people in this world only think of theirselves.

bridgett

I found pictures of women who had mastectomies and found one that had a tattoo on her chest wall around the scar. I asked my husband what he thought about a tattoo. He did not think that was a good idea—he loves me just the way I am—and I have had enough done to my chest.

memphisgirl

Shyness and modesty

Having a reconstructed breast has its own set of problems but I am very shy. I do not like drawing attention to myself in any way and even though most people are polite, I didn't like everyone noticing this. If anything, I think people feel sorry for you. I was physically very comfortable without a breast prior to my reconstruction and there was this side of me that just wanted to say to the world, "This happened to me so deal with it because I don't want to hide." But some courage just takes too much energy. I really admire the women who can do it though.

ScaredSilly

My greatest wish is to be confident enough to do without the prosthesis. I worry so much about the reactions of others. I know that is the wrong approach, but it is the best I can do right now. I do have a safe zone (home, immediate neighborhood for walking, family, and a few close friends). However, every situation requires careful consideration as to what I must wear. Winter is easier with multiple layers. I also exercise and have worked out a system to change in the gym (I will *not* go into the little closet set aside for the people like me!).

cj

I am a person who has always been modest about my body. I had large breasts and did everything I could to hide them. I always joke that I was given a Godsmack for being so self-conscious. I have had to bare my breasts to so many people throughout this cancer journey. Even though I currently have one breast and another with just a tissue expander, I am not self-conscious anymore. I feel that cancer allowed me to be self-forgiving of perceived body flaws. I look at all of my scars as chapters in the great journey that I have been on.

Lauren

The first thing you have to lose when you have been diagnosed with breast cancer is your modesty. That is something that goes right out the window. Your breasts are pinched, probed, then cut on, molded, painted, burned, and put on display for all the medical world to see. So if you have a problem with modesty you better get over it. I did.

Jackjoy

I was 18 when my mother was diagnosed with breast cancer. For the five years she was alive I never saw her undressed or without her bra and prosthesis. It was all a mystery to me. Even the word *cancer* was never spoken out loud. It is now 35 years later. How things have changed. I am very open about my surgery, my chest—or lack of one—and my prosthesis. For me, it is the only way to be.

smilie

CHAPTER SEVEN

Love Relationships and Sexual Intimacy

"A healthy sex life is part of life."

zoochild

T*he women had so much to say about love and intimacy that our early versions of this chapter would have filled up half of this book. What does that suggest? For one thing, this is a topic that women with breast cancer need to communicate about; romantic love and connecting sexually is of great importance* especially *when coping with breast cancer; and being a "good girl" and keeping your feelings to yourself is no longer an acceptable option. To quote an old cliché, it's not that we have "sex on the brain"—to the contrary. As one woman states, "I have always believed your brain is your biggest sex organ."*

Once you "mess" with a woman's breast, the sexual implications are tremendous; add to that the necessary medicine to combat further disease and you are now affecting a woman's internal "ecosystem," often resulting in changes that for her are unforeseen, unexplained, and little understood. Tell an actively sexual thirty-year-old that she will be going into menopause and you will get a blank stare in reply; once it happens, though, she will have aged in ways far vaster than any of her sexual organs have. And what about feeling desirable? Or holding a marriage together as each of you struggles with change? For those of you who are single—for whatever reasons—dating can be as much fun as swatting away flies at a picnic. There are plenty of jokes and wry comments here (worrying about your wig staying on when you kiss; trying to read the instructions for myriad lubricants in the dark) because laughter is healthy medicine—and it's organic, too!

Sometimes the honesty took my breath away: women discuss being sexually abused, not having had sex for years, deeply missing their breasts when making love. They speak of the tender ways in which a spouse helped to bathe and take care of them and how cuddling comes to replace active lovemaking. I suppose this is our R-rated chapter, for the anecdotes and advice are often graphic and explicit. Sex and sexuality, libido and desire, even masturbation are part of the yeasty and complex components of loving relationships, and they're all discussed here. Communication is like the keyboard upon which the emotional and physical notes are played, because "it's not just sex, it's our whole relationships that have changed." No doubt about it: these women are charting new ground as they lay out the terrain of sexual love for those with breast cancer. With all the effort and thought and desire that go into loving relationships, we are left asking ourselves this: If intimacy is so essential and love takes many forms, why is it so hard to achieve?

THE BIG PICTURE

"We are too young to have our sexuality taken from us. Relationships are hard enough, but tell a man you feel you could go the rest of your life without sex and see the response you get!"

Gila

If a man stops loving you because of the way your chest looks he is definitely not worth it. I am very honest about having had breast cancer. I tell everyone, even 8 years later. It was and still is part of my life.

    Joanne

When I was first diagnosed and before my surgery I would cry after sex thinking I was going to be changed and that my husband would see me differently. But thank God for good men—he has been wonderful. It just took me time to get through all the emotional turmoil I was experiencing.

    Terry

> "I had fears about my scars, etc., but believe they tell stories and should be shared with the one I love."
>
>   Greatful2b

I have been divorced for 8 years and have not had sex for 9. I would like to have a loving relationship with someone, but have not met any single men my age that even offered the slightest interest in me as a woman. The mastectomy just further entrenched the possibility that I may be single for the rest of my life. This offers a possibility that another relationship could develop out of friendship, even if attraction is not the catalyst. There are good men out there . . . but are any of them single?

    Isurrender

> "Sometimes I think my only problem in life was being born female."
>
>   Delivered

"I am a walking billboard for the fact that there is life after a mastectomy."

Mary Pat

My need for closeness, hugs, warm smiles, hand holding have increased while my sex drive has decreased. I think about having sex, but I'm just too tired or uncomfortable most of the time. When it does happen, I am extremely aware of what parts are missing and feel myself tighten up when he gets near.

stillhealing

"The vagina is a very forgiving organ."

abrenner

I am often scared to be in love, whether it is with my husband or my 3 children. The fear of getting seriously ill again at times can be paralyzing. This was the case for me in the early years after my diagnosis. Over time, I have learned to trust more, but you never forget the road you traveled. I never want to see my family endure another serious illness with me, at least not for a long, long time. I sometimes associate love with loss. It's crazy, but I think that's what my breast cancer experience may have brought up for me as it relates to my relationships. I may be way ahead of myself and my worry sometimes gets the best of me.

Eileen

"Cancer can either make or break a relationship. If it wasn't good to begin with, cancer sure isn't going to help."

BCWarrior

I keep going back to the idea of toxic people and tonic people. Definitely ditching the former is a good thing even if it means less nookie.
    MCN

At times, I believe I was so focused on my own mortality and life that I often forgot about his fears too.
    LaurieV

At age 22 I lost both breasts. I am 58 now. It has been so long, I often wonder what a breast feels like. I look at women and wonder what it would feel like to touch their breast, to feel a nipple. Not that I desire women sexually, I just want to feel a natural breast. I am a woman, a mother, and I haven't felt or seen natural breasts for 36 years. I miss them.
    kathynye

I swear, I am a walking billboard for the fact that there is life after a mastectomy. When my fiancé walked out on me after my second chemo, I thought it was worse than the diagnosis. Everyone said he did you a favor because he was a rat. I didn't feel that way at the time. I suffered so my skin hurt, I so missed the touching. It was such a rough year because I read all the BS about positive thinking and I was so devastated by losing him, that I was afraid I wasn't thinking positive, so I would have a recurrence, blah blah blah. I look back at my 14 years since then and I can't believe all of my experiences with men.

It was the first time in my life I was alone, I didn't have kids home anymore, they were all in or out of college, but I was still young. I live in a golf resort community and I met some great men; one said, as I warned him I had a problem, that he was worried I was going to say I had herpes. Another loved my botched-up reconstructed breast the best. He said it was his favorite because it was so brave. I could go on but can't allow myself to think too much about ten years of being somewhat slutty since I am now married for three years and my husband would be shocked to know my past.

I had affairs with married men, one a U.S. Congressman, major CEOs, lawyers, hot shots, a good-looking young surfer who said if it came back, he would just take me to all the beaches in the world, and never once had anyone reject me because of the cancer. I think now it was sick of me trying to prove myself appealing. But it sure was fun.

My point is sexuality is not body parts. Men love us for our essence. There sure are some great guys out there and I wish every one of you find one or keep the one you have, who will love you for who you are, just the way you are.

Mary Pat

YOUR BODY IMAGE—THE GOOD, THE BAD, AND THE IN-BETWEEN

> "My body has been through a lot. But it's the only one I got and I have to do the best with what I have."
>
> kathynye

Perhaps it's because I'm in a committed relationship with someone who knew me before cancer and its resulting scars that I am not afraid of intimacy. Sure, there was initially some concern that the physical reality might somehow become a barrier, that my body would get in the way of my essence and I would be less desirable, but that's not happened. In the years since my cancer my partner has had prostate cancer and gall bladder surgeries of his own so it's not like either one of us is unscarred. That caused us to become more creative in our sexual intimacy. We both find that scarred bodies are somehow more real, tested, and certain.

Susan

I haven't been in a sexual relationship for about 10 years. (Wow! That seems really long after seeing it in print!) The last relationship ended at my insistence because I was feeling used and had realized that there was no real future for us. With my history of childhood sexual abuse, I always had trouble setting boundaries where sex was concerned, and had ended up in a bad marriage and a long-term relationship with an alcoholic. In spite of the childhood abuse, I've always enjoyed sex. However, I decided there would be no more sex until I was married again. Since I also have problems with intimacy (with anyone) at times, that hasn't happened. Sometimes I really miss that. Sometimes I'm very grateful that the desire has decreased (for quite a while it was nonexistent). Mostly I have a "wait and see" attitude: if it happens, fantastic, if not, that's okay.

HopeNFaith

I've had problems since my double mastectomy and reconstruction followed by chemo and radiation (2½ years ago at age 53). My husband of 35 years is soooo patient, but I'm easily frustrated because my body won't work like it used to. The chemo caused "chemopause." I can't see myself as physically desirable because of these fake, do-nothing boobs. I know my "bad thinking" isn't helping. Just can't get my head on straight. I sometimes cry quietly when we finish with sex because it used to be more than wonderful, and now it's . . . not. In addition to the boob problem, my gynecologist explained sex is very painful for me because the lack of hormones have caused what was the hymen tissues to shrink and lose elasticity making penetration extremely painful and impossible. In a normal menopause the hormones change gradually over a longer time frame, but mine changed in just a few weeks. So in the sex department I feel like

I'm missing a lot. I'm working on a better attitude, if not a more satisfied sex life.

Bach

I chose tram-flap reconstruction, so have only tactile feeling in my breasts and reduced feeling in my abdomen area. Although the mastectomies were complete, there was no need for radiation or chemo, and after much discussion with my doctors, I began taking hormone replacement again. Without HRT, I had dryness and basically no interest in sex whatsoever. When I was diagnosed with breast cancer, I was in a relationship. He was terrific during my surgeries, but did not want me to have reconstruction. However, I was determined to have the reconstruction for me, so I would not marry him until after that surgery. I gave him plenty of opportunity to change his mind if this was all too much for him. He didn't. I had the reconstruction in May and we got married in July. He was overly cautious for a long time, but finally I think we are back on the right track, sexually. Even though I don't have feeling in my breasts, I know when they are being touched, at least in a general way. I thought sexual feelings were mostly mental, but when I was not taking HRT, I really didn't have any interest. I like those hormones.

Al

I also think that part of me doesn't want to think about sex or starting a new relationship because then I would have to deal with the issue of what will any guy think of me with only one "real" boob and one reconstructed boob. It is hard for me to open myself up to others and the possibility of rejection.

suzie

I have one real and one no-boob, having elected not to reconstruct. Then I kicked out my husband and now wonder if a man would find me "acceptable." I have been reassured by a friend that they are out there as she met her husband after a complete (not partial) mastectomy. Libido is gone, but I figure we're alive, wonderful, and eventually will find our ways back to passion.

Juneboomer

THE OLD ME VS. THE NEW ME: OVERWEIGHT, NO SEX DRIVE, JUST PLAIN TIRED

Everything in the area of sex has been turned upside down for me. Before cancer and treatment, I was a healthy, sexually vibrant 44-year-old who really enjoyed sex with her husband. Now, two years later, I am 15 pounds overweight, I have almost continuous hot flashes, and I have little to no desire for sex. I feel as though my husband wishes that he could have the "old me" back because his passion for me is totally gone. This has been almost harder for me to deal with than the actual cancer because it has taken such a toll on our marriage. I feel as though my body has aged 20 years in a short period of time, and that I am trapped inside!

Lizzie Lou

> "The hardest part for me is every time we make love I think about the cancer the entire time and I am tired of thinking about it."
>
> Alix

Sometimes I think my only problem in life was being born female. Truly though, I think the only reason I have any concern over my body image (weight, scarring, etc.) is because I want to give my hubby the best. The problem is that I have not yet accepted the current version of me as the final definition of *my* best. Hmmm. Okay, guess I just turned on my own light bulb. I'm gonna get up off my chubby tush and do something about it. I don't have to be a movie-star model, but I really think I can get a little healthier looking than what I'm seeing in the mirror.

Delivered

FEELING DESIRABLE

This experience has been tough for me. I hope as time passes I will feel better about myself. My husband of 13 years has been so supportive and caring. He loves all of me. While that is such a tremendous relief, I am the one with the problem. Right now I'm bald, have 2 incisions across my chest, and have gained 20 pounds. I'm not feeling very pretty or desirable. I'm still very emotional about all this and it just makes me cry. Intimacy is so important and I find myself pulling away more because of my own stupid low self-image.

Beth's still smiling

> "I want to be close. I want to be loved. But I don't really want to have sex. I wish I felt as good about me as my husband does."
>
> Delivered

It was very important to me to resume intimacy with my husband as soon as possible after the surgery; I had to know that I was still appealing to him. I think all of this lopsidedness and scars matter a lot more to me than it does to him.

Nett

I feel that so much has happened to me over the past two years, and my husband has had to do soooo much for me (nursing, cleaning, etc.) I couldn't possibly be lovable. He's seen me at my absolute worst! But

I've had to do similar things for my son and grandson as well as my husband and I certainly love them. They are lovable, so why shouldn't I be lovable too? I still have a need for intimacy, but I no longer initiate it. I guess I'm afraid of rejection. I sometimes feel that I'm contaminated. This disease and treatment has really done a number on me. I don't know what to do or how to think most of the time.

Blessed

I had never worried about being lovable until I had my daughter. It took a long time for my husband to perceive me as a lover and sexy again after she came along (c-section and then I nursed her for a year). When I found my lump I worried that my husband would never be able to reconcile the changes that I knew I needed to make physically in order to give myself the best possible outcome. And I was right. It has been five years, and he still has a hard time touching me, touching my reconstructed breasts, or even thinking of me in sexual ways. We didn't have sex at all for 13 months after my surgery. We now have relations, somewhat regularly, but the passion, or what there ever was of it, is gone.

Suffice it to say that I was a hottie sexually when I met my husband, and we were doing okay after the baby. But not since I got sick. Some of it is that I don't feel sexy at all anymore. Not because of the way my husband feels, or because I've gained weight, but because I don't really like the way I look. My husband and I are very committed to our relationship and staying together. I just hope that in time we can find a way to help ourselves find comfort in each other that can translate into physical desire and love.

abrenner

I am a rather tall, thin woman who never had breasts that would be considered large in any way, shape or form. My husband never complained, so I didn't worry! Anyway, on to my feelings about being lovable after surgery: No! A thousand times no! I didn't feel lovable at all and did not want my husband to see me during intimate times. Although he had helped me shower when the drains were still in and done all sorts of caretaking measures, I did not want him to have to experience me as I was when we were being close. Oh God, I felt so bad then. Perhaps that had something to do with our separation. Who knows? We still found ways to satisfy one another but it was never the same for me and, I suppose, never the same for him either.

Intimacy changed so drastically then. I wanted to be held and caressed and fondled. He wanted *sex*! We never spoke of the changes and by the time I realized that we should be speaking of them, it was too late. He had opted me out of his life.

After over two years since the separation, I feel more secure about my body now. But I don't think that I could ever be close to anyone again. I would pull away in fear of a re-hash of my marriage breakup. Not worthy, etc. This part of my life was and is a mess. Yikes! Just talking about it here makes me see that I have a definite problem.

Ladyblue930

I was never confident of my femininity or sexuality, even during my 23-year marriage. Now, at a time when my sons are grown and I would like to find a loving relationship, I feel very poorly equipped to attract a man. I never gave it much importance before, and now find myself wondering how to balance the reality of my situation against my beliefs that it shouldn't count.

Isurrender

Worry about being lovable? *You betcha!!*
Scared to be in love (or stay in love)? *Yes.*
Need for intimacy? *What's that?*
Minefield of complex feelings? *Yes again!*
Addressed the feelings? *No.*

carolecare

MARRIAGE

What a roller coaster marriage is—and that's when you're both healthy! Pact (your wedding vows) and impact (your disease): whether it's at the breakfast table or in the privacy of your bedroom, the commitments you originally made to one another undergo change and, hopefully, renewal.

A minefield of complex feelings

I have learned to enjoy what I can. It has made my husband feel "what's the use?" since he knows that he can't give me full satisfaction. He has considered having an affair, which I knew was coming. And he hasn't. Talking it out, not just once, but many times, has helped keep our marriage together.

jennagram

> "I have always believed that your brain is your biggest sex organ."
>
> jjensen

I feel like sexual intimacy has become a minefield of complex feelings for me. I was originally diagnosed with Stage II breast cancer 5 years ago and had a Stage IV recurrence 1 year ago. Whenever my health was bad, sex and intimacy would make me cry, then my husband would cry too. This was not my idea of fun sex, but I couldn't help it. We have been together for 24 years and have grown closer and worked through the emotions, but intimacy seems to bring all of the fears to the surface for me.

BandMom46

I am 44 and was very active sexually with my husband before cancer 3 years ago. I think at first it was a little fear, then it was lack of desire.

Now I'm not sure what it is. The physical part just isn't there often. I wonder if it is partly the tamoxifen. It also is my husband—he doesn't approach me as much either.

tinkr59bell

> "We love each other more than ever, but sex sure isn't as fun as it was before cancer."
>
> BandMom46

My marriage (28 years) has not been the best. Many times over the years I have contemplated divorce. A lot of the time my husband was inattentive, rude, and sometimes even cruel. Optimistic me just kept thinking it would get better. When my son died, almost nine years ago, I fell apart. I just didn't care anymore. I tried, but could not let go of my mourning. When I finally—over five years later—began coming out of my funk, my husband and I began growing closer. For the next two years it was as if we were getting to know each other again. Then I was diagnosed with cancer. I am proud to say he has not left my side for any test or appointment. He used to not speak to me for days if I cried. Now he holds me and when appropriate makes jokes to get me laughing.

I share all this with you because now I will tell you that I, too, have no sexual drive. When my husband would enter me it would hurt so badly that sometimes I would cry. And when he ejaculated it felt like liquid fire. But I still so wanted the intimacy—the touching of naked bodies, the kissing and exploring. Believe it or not, he came up with the answer. We use rubbers! And Astroglide! And you can't imagine how much better it is. Once we get past the entry, it's okay. I always try and make the slipping on of the condom very special. Role play, ladies. Make it special in new ways that fit what you have to work with. Sometimes it is so very difficult, but together we are trying to make the very best of what we have and I am just so very thankful. I have never felt so loved or special.

San

I come from a very conservative background and always got dressed in the closet so my husband would not see me naked. Every morning for years he would try to peek in and catch me in various stages of undress—it was fun, it was silly, it was sexy. After my bilateral mastectomy he stopped looking. I was crushed; I felt like damaged goods. It was not until we were at the brink of divorce and seeing a marriage counselor that I learned that he stopped our silly little ritual because he thought it would make me feel bad if he continued to try to see me naked after my breasts were gone. He was trying to protect my feelings and I misunderstood his action and didn't ask. We are still struggling.

SandyF

Marriage and intimacy: "to have and to hold"

I am 55 and I tell you this because it is possible my age has something to do with my attitude. Twelve years ago I had a complete hysterectomy so that was when I first encountered lack of lubrication and elasticity. I was already having difficulty with intercourse before my surgery. And since the surgery my desire for intercourse has dropped to zero. However, I am very lucky that the lack of sex has not caused any strain in my marriage. My husband and I have been through so many other losses and sex is such a small issue in comparison. My dear husband keeps telling me that having me alive and by his side is more important than sex. We are still very intimate. We kiss and touch, snuggle on the sofa, enjoy spending time together, and love each other more every day. However we do wish that sex wasn't so much work when we do decide to go for it.

clk913

We've been married for 33 years and my husband has stood by me through lots of stuff, including this cancer mess. He never had any issues with my lopsidedness; it's been hard for him this second time around with the Stage IV cancer. We're both 65 and the meds that I have been on (aromatase inhibitors) have reduced my libido to zip. But I still want to be intimate with him. We both still love cuddling and we do that every night before we fall asleep. He has taught me that it is not the sex that counts so much as the tenderness and expression of loving feelings. And the worst fear I have with the cancer is dying before he does and thinking of how lonely he will be. I have to stop thinking that way, though. One day at a time, right?

Annie Mac

We never referred to it as sex; it was always making love and part of making love is the holding and caressing and the closeness we get from being with that other person. So now making love is not the actual intercourse but everything that leads up to it and everything after, including falling asleep and waking each morning with that person. So actually my sex drive was never parked because he was always there to hold me and kiss me and comfort me and if it led to more then that was great; if not it was just as great because we always had each other and we still do. If anything, cancer has brought us closer without having to have intercourse.

lilybelle2

After my mastectomy, I would ask my husband if it [sex] was really awful and did it change how he felt about me, etc. His response: "Actually, it's kind of exotic." He's not one to mince words or say things to be nice, so this was genuine. Going through breast cancer brought us much closer together. Without his support and continued support, I don't know what I would have done.

Annie

I am also fortunate in that my husband has been attentive and loving and supportive. We've had our share of difficulties, though, when it comes to sexual intimacy.

I have found that I just don't seem to have much sex drive or desire. It used to be that if we didn't make love pretty regularly, I would have erotic dreams and even have orgasms as a result. But that has only happened once or twice in the past 6 months. It takes longer for me to get aroused. And I haven't had an orgasm like I used to. Unfortunately, having no breasts is harder for me than my husband when it comes to sexual intimacy. Stimulation of my breasts and nipples was nice for him but incredibly arousing for me and almost always led to powerful orgasms. We have been unable to find a "substitute" for that sensation.

My husband is very reassuring and loving; both his words and actions let me know that he still thinks I'm sexy. But I don't feel sexy, and sometimes I feel really ugly. We talk and hold each other close, and I know he will be patient as we work through this, but sometimes I get so angry because our sex life was terrific and it isn't anymore. I don't know if it will be again.

We both sleep in the nude, but when we make love I wear a camisole or a T-shirt. I'm not ready for my breastless-ness to be "right there" when we make love.

kamaha

Scarcity of sex in the marriage

My husband (of 28 years) and I have not yet gotten back the physical part of our relationship. We're closer than ever emotionally and do not fight at all, but he hasn't gotten used to my new body, the scars and weight gain. We haven't given up yet, but it is hard. We're too young to have stopped having intercourse.

mtn woman

Mtn woman,

Keep fighting to gain control over your sex life. It's worth the fight. I wait until my husband is sleepy and it's dark in the room (he can't really see the scars and weight gain). Back rub usually leads to other parts being rubbed and then he is ready for sex. Good luck!

connie

My sex drive has left the building and when it returns for a small showing it always seems to be when my husband is not ready, e.g., it's too early, the kids could come in, he's tired. Boy, I thought I would never hear some of those words out of his mouth. I am trying to get my meds adjusted so I can get a real sex drive with passion and everything that goes with it. I had a great recon as well tram flap both sides, but he knows that they don't feel the same for me anymore and he doesn't enjoy them like he used to. It's funny that I can't enjoy the sun like I used to (skin cancer), can't enjoy sex like I used to (no drive/pain/dryness). So I look like a cut-up, pale, wrinkled ole plump woman that even in my dreams—and this is true—a guy refused to rape me because I looked so hideous.

Mel

The challenges of married life for those under forty

Your twenties and thirties are the years when you glow—your skin is smooth and moist, your hair is plentiful, and your mind is sharp. And . . . you are sexually active, physically and emotionally. With one fell swoop, breast cancer for those not yet forty can undo all of that.

"In almost 3 years since my mastectomy,
I have never had sex with my shirt off."

BCWarrior

In all honesty, just before breast cancer my libido was waning already—we had 3 kids under 4 at that point. Now the kids are more grown and not wearing me out so much, but where is my sex drive? I'll be 3 years out this September and I (and my husband) have been cutting me much slack. I'm not sure how to approach it but have talked to a psychotherapist about it. She said I shouldn't be so hard on myself. At what point should I try harder? And what should I try? I usually put off his advances and he doesn't force the issue, and then I feel guilty. We tried watching porn a few times which got me going a bit (but what a crutch!) and it got him too excited so he went way too fast (then he felt bad and now worries he won't perform)! I guess we are lucky that we are best friends as well as lovers, but I'd like to get the sex thing figured out. We are kind of a mess.

    Anne M.

I really love sex. It was rough during treatment when I lost my libido due to menopause. Things came back slowly though; my husband is very understanding. Fortunately for me he was never a "boob man." One thing that has changed though: in almost 3 years since my mastectomy, I have never had sex with my shirt off. I don't think either of us is comfortable with it. But so what? My remaining breast is saggy from children so I guess I'd be self-conscious anyway :)

    BCWarrior

I also won't have sex without a shirt on and I always ask if he wants me to put my other breast on so he can have two to touch. He always says no.

    april 4 us

I was enjoying my sex life very much and since my husband is 8 years younger than me he always had a high sex drive. The chemo put me in menopause and the tamoxifen keeps me there. I have absolutely no desire for sex anymore but pretend that I do for my husband's sake. I have to use KY Jelly and now get frequent yeast infections because of the dryness problem. My husband is wonderful and patient and when I comment on all of my scars making me look like Frankenstein he gets mad at me and tells me that I am still beautiful. We do still cuddle a lot and spoon in bed so we always have the sexual connection, we just don't always make love. I don't think that my self-esteem would be as intact if I did not have him. We have a great relationship and friendship. Besides, it's hard to have a sex life with two teenagers in the house!

   flower girl

If truth be told, I feel sorry for my husband because he is a 32-year-old man who has had to learn all the ins and outs of breast cancer. I know that marriage is in sickness and in health but I just wish we didn't have to face the sickness part so soon.

   Lauren

THE DATING GAME: SINGLE AND DATING

Tick-tock, tick-tock: is there a so-called right time to tell someone you're dating that you've had breast cancer?

> "I know that casual sex will never be an option for me."
>
>   reginabu

I am single and have not been with any man since I had my bilateral mastectomy. I don't intend to tell a man on the first date that I've been "rebuilt." When do you think it's the right time to tell him? Obviously if I sense it bothers him, he's not the right man for me. If the relationship proceeds to intimacy, I am petrified about him seeing me and about my lack of sensation. I can't believe I'll be much of an intimate partner.

Flamingo

Flamingo,

I think when you allow the right person to come into your personal space then and only then will you feel it's the right time; I don't know that that's something that another person could tell you. And you are right about our bodies being rebuilt. I also have not been with anyone since my diagnosis and even before that I was practicing celibacy for about three years. I would love to find myself in a relationship someday soon but I've been so tied up with my cancer thing (smile) and trying to keep myself in a good peaceful frame of mind that I guess I haven't been thinking about it much. I think more men should join these types of forums so that they can be more in tune to what women are really thinking and feeling. Do you think that would help them understand us more?

river

> "In some ways my cancer has been a blessing. I have found a truly wonderful man; if it weren't for cancer I might not have noticed how special he really is."
>
> nikko

I was wondering if anyone else had the problem of when to tell a guy that you are a breast cancer survivor?? I used to tell them right away to get it out of the way since it was always on my mind anyway. I figured it out that it was too soon and it was scaring the guys off! So now I don't know exactly what to do. I feel like being a cancer survivor defines me so much that I need to share that info, but I don't want to share that info too soon. I have a scar from a lumpectomy so I need to probably tell before any sexual contact happens. I don't know; I am confused about what to do now. Not that I have a whole lot of dates anyway, but it happens once in a while!

Suzette

ScaredSilly is indeed scared to tell a man she has cancer; RC is just the opposite

I worry about telling a new man that I have cancer. I do not want to see the look on his face at that time. I am 55 and most people at this age are looking forward to enjoying retirement and don't want to be burdened with a sick person. My latest interest just finished caring for a wife of 29 years who had MS. He made the remark that he is looking forward to having his life back. How do I tell him I've had Stage III cancer and 20 lymph nodes removed. If the situation was reversed I think I would opt out.

ScaredSilly

I had been casually dating a fellow, about every 3 weeks or so, for about 4 months before I was diagnosed. My children were not home one Sunday AM, so I called and asked him to come by for coffee. This was difficult for him because he is not very good at impromptu. I ended up saying "it is not a big deal, just a few moments for coffee." He came by before I could even serve the coffee. I let him know I had cancer so I would be busy for a while. He didn't quite understand. I ended up saying, "Look, I am going to be bald!" He just said "Oh, I loved that movie with Sigourney Weaver when she was bald." I thought he was just out of his mind! Anyway, we still date (3½ years later). I would have never imagined.

My lesson in that is there truly are non-judgmental people. It has also taught me not to accept anything less. We did not start a sexual relationship until I was bald. That was very comforting during that time. I think it really helped my self-esteem. I look back and am grateful to have had that. We started seeing each other once a week after I had told him and he would always come by the evening I had chemo and just lay with me. Both of us are fiercely independent, so neither would be "burdened" concerning my health issues. That is not how our relationship is structured.

ScaredSilly, do not be afraid; take the chance if it arises. If things don't go well consider yourself "saved from an asshole" and move on!

RC

I told my new beau about the cancer last night. He was very good about it and made a remark that made me think he did not see this as a deal breaker. I think he likes me. He called this morning to ask how I was feeling and wanted to make sure I hadn't gotten too tired out. I don't want everything to be about my cancer, however. I think with enough conversations we can get to a good place.

ScaredSilly

Being single is hard. You wonder if anyone can or will love you someday. Knowing that you are sick, you wonder what they will think if and when they see your body as it is now. Can they get past it and have sex not looking or thinking about the scars? At least there is one consolation: if a man does fall in love with you, you know it is for who you are! Still it scares me: will I ever love and be loved?

SacredHeart

After the end of treatment, I just by chance met someone who was interested in me, not knowing what I had been through. I was still wearing a wig and absolutely terrified to go on a date, wondering how I could possibly tell him all this and imagining him running screaming out the door. I thought I would just go on one date to get out a bit. But then he wanted to see me again. What's a girl to do?? It was actually quite comical, because the first time he tried to kiss me, I had to stop him and get through the entire story—the cancer, the wig (couldn't let the wig fall off on the first kiss!!). And he was so wonderful about it, and actually encouraged me to take off the wig. I think by the time I got around to the cancer part, he was just so relieved I wasn't giving him the boot. I never expected to have someone help me through that most difficult time and make me feel desirable. That was a true gift. And while he's no longer around, I will always be thankful for what he did for me.

Even though the scars are healed now, I still find it difficult at the start of a relationship to figure out when to talk about my illness. I have the fear, not of my sexuality or desirability, but that the other person won't want to be with me long-term because of the implications of my illness. If anything, the experience of cancer has made my physical experiences deeper and more meaningful, but my fears greater.

    Nushka

I have been very fortunate. I had just started dating a new man a few weeks before being diagnosed with breast cancer; I was afraid to tell him I was having a biopsy thinking he would run for the hills. Instead the complete opposite happened. It pulled us together and we have become very close. If it weren't for my cancer we would probably still be trying to decide whether or not we wanted to continue seeing each other. Instead we are madly in love! In the beginning I did make a determination to be the most inspirational cancer patient ever and I shared this determination with my boyfriend. I've had my lumpectomy and am just getting ready to start radiation in 2 weeks.

In some ways my cancer has been a blessing. I have found a truly wonderful man; if it weren't for cancer I might not have noticed how special he really is.

    nikko

I've been without anyone for 6 or 7 years and have forgotten completely what sex is about. Mostly, I want a man to be my best friend, so sex is on the back burner for me. So maybe my libido is also in the toilet, not sure. Probably because sex might lead to pregnancy which might lead to a recurrence, although I've been encouraged by so many I hear getting pregnant after treatment. I've decided not to get reconstruction which I'm okay with, but I don't know anyone my size, a C cup, of my age who doesn't get reconstruction. Is everyone getting it so that guys will find them attractive? I guess I'm not sure what's better: having a husband who you've had great sex with and now feel like it's not so great, or me—hopefully meeting someone some day, and them not knowing how great it could have been. I just know that I'll tell that first guy, "Do you know how great-looking my boobs were!"

moxie

In September of 2002, moxie was diagnosed with Stage III breast cancer, two years to the day that her mother died from the disease.

The idea of figuring out when and how to tell someone is a tough one that is relevant to me this very week since I've been on several dates with a lovely man who knows I've had cancer but doesn't yet know that I've had a mastectomy. This has been my first dating experience in over a year and is my first experience post–breast cancer.

I'm finding that I'm more hesitant and physically shy even about kissing, although part of that may come from osmosis from being surrounded by Islamic morality here in the Gulf that doesn't go for public displays of affection.* Even so, I dread what the make-over shows would call "the reveal" and I have no idea how he'll take it.

I envy those of you who have a life partner who has seen you through this. Even if a man accepts me for everything I am (and I have no reason to think one won't), he won't ever really "get it." I feel a loss at not having that intimacy with someone who was there to shave my head and kiss my stitches, laugh at my wild gypsy scarf and feel me up one last time before surgery. My hope is to find someone who is the sort of person that would have been there had we known each other. If not, then I hope to stay sassy and strong on my own.

MCN

MCN lives outside of Dubai, where she teaches Arab women to be primary-school English teachers. She was diagnosed while there at the age of thirty-one.

Becoming involved when you are living with advanced-stage breast cancer

I am single and had a boyfriend when I was first diagnosed (had just turned 40) who was very understanding (I think he actually liked the reconstruction period where I had one huge boob during the time they were stretching my skin). I went with several men after that and each time before even getting to the intimacy stage, I felt compelled to say, "Umm, there is something you better know about me." None of them ran away or were shocked, as I expected they would be. Then I had a recurrence and was diagnosed as Stage IV and it was even a bigger problem.

I met someone I really liked, but before we got serious I had to tell him, I have had a mastectomy and I had reconstruction, but the problem is I didn't just have breast cancer, I *have* it and it isn't going to go away and I don't know what is going to happen because I have only been on treatment for a few months. (I talk like that—am queen of the run-on sentence they tell me.) Anyway, we went on to date, got engaged, and lived together for three years. The hormonal treatments threw me into menopause and I am totally dried up. I am now dating someone I went to high school with and he's very understanding about my lack of interest in sex as well as the discomfort it causes me when we do try to do it, perhaps because he is 55 years old also and maybe he's thankful to have a woman who isn't demanding, someone he doesn't have to worry about satisfying.

Anyway, I find it absolutely amazing how little having boobs means to a man if he is really interested in you; shows that men are not nearly as shallow as I thought they were and it was in fact me who was the shallow thinker.

I don't really miss sex, but do miss the feeling of intimacy that went with it, however that is another one of my mental issues—am not able to really commit to a relationship and totally back away and put up my fence when it gets too involved.

Marybe

Happily single

I'm single and was without a partner when I was diagnosed. I find I'm now completely and totally uninterested in sex and/or intimacy and it's been a year and a half since I finished treatment. Most of you seem to be married so you can hardly ignore the lack of desire the way I can. Part of the problem is my weight and part of it's my hating the way I look now. The rest is probably the total lack of estrogen (had both ovaries removed 3 weeks after my breast surgery). I've decided to just accept this is where I am and go about reclaiming the rest of my life by getting back in shape, traveling, and doing everything and anything I've ever wanted to—except date or have sex. I know this probably sounds terrible to you, but I'm actually feeling pretty good about myself otherwise.

pennywise

Pennywise, I'm married for almost 11 years (2nd marriage) and I can tell you that for me, what you wrote about not being interested in dating or having sex does not sound terrible or even weird to me at all. Focusing on yourself, putting your new life together; these are really important things to do for yourself post-treatment, in my opinion. I consider you *lucky*. You have the time and freedom to focus on yourself without having to worry about a partner or child.

I'm not saying that those of us who are partnered or parents are not lucky. I'm trying to say that there are times when it would be great to be able to focus on just me. Finding myself. Rediscovering and making peace with my body. Figuring out how to reclaim my life, as Pennywise says, or "owning" the life I've now been thrust into from my breast cancer experience, without having to worry in any way about anyone else. That was the part of single life that I must admit I really do miss. I love my family, but I also loved not having to "be" for anyone else but me.

abrenner

DIVORCED AND DATING

Since I've been celibate for over three years, this is a tough one. I think breast cancer would have had a huge effect if I was still married to my ex. Sex was the top priority for him, even after 18 years of marriage. Dealing with his reaction to all of this would have been more devastating than the breast cancer itself. I still feel lovable, and started dating someone during chemo, though it turned out to be a short-term relationship. We never got to the point where intimacy was an issue, but, yeah, I worried about it. We met via the Internet, so my main concern was about how much to tell him and when. I wasn't comfortable with being deceptive or dishonest about the whole thing. What if I said nothing, and my wig blew off or something? So, before we met, I sent him an e-mail telling him I was being treated for cancer and was wearing a wig. I also mentioned my cosmetically enhanced eyebrows. His response was that it wasn't a big deal, because none of us are perfect. Over the next three dates we discussed exactly what kind of cancer and treatment I'd had, and he seemed fine with it. Anyway, I got the first date in more than 20 years over with and survived.

My biggest concern about a serious relationship or remarriage isn't so much to do with intimacy and sex as it is about the uncertainty of the future. If someone my age is looking for a "life partner," they won't be looking for someone whose life expectancy is questionable. And I don't know that it would be fair of me to ask someone to plan a future with me that may be nothing more than wishful thinking. I just plan to wait and see what God has in store for me. If that special someone is out there, I'll meet him when the time is right. If not, I'm perfectly happy on my own.

    kathi1964

I am also single by choice for now. I was married for 20 years and have been divorced for about eight years now. After I was diagnosed, most of my energy has been spent making sure I stay healthy and happy. Although I'd like to be married again I decided not to push it. I do think that if you meet someone that you are really interested in you should have that talk with them, however not everyone that you'll meet will need to know. I've learned that not every dinner and a movie a relationship makes. I strongly agree with you: I feel like I am and will be defined as a cancer survivor and somewhat judged.

    river

When you are single and hit with breast cancer, it sure is tough. It is challenging enough to be 50, a woman without a partner, but when you are a breast cancer survivor with the health and sexual issues, it seems like another tall mountain to climb.

    mspet

I just celebrated my 30th birthday. The thought of finding someone to take on a relationship with me and my 3-year-old is bad enough without now having to add the burden of my struggles and the baggage that comes with it. Every day I get out of the shower, I stare at myself in the mirror and think, If I can't look at myself, how can I ever expect anyone else to? I know that I am still so young and have so much to be thankful for. So why can't I get past all this sadness?

    kw4184

WIDOWED AND DATING

I'm a widow and have begun thinking of socializing again and perhaps dating. I'm going to start with a widows/widowers social group in a suburb about 10 miles from where I live, my theory being it will be a "safe" group who've gone through the grief experience and the likelihood that I will know someone is remote, sort of starting with a clean slate. My kids, thankfully, are pushing me to begin dating again; they think I'm too young at 56 to be alone the rest of my life. So a new adventure begins. Don't you just love these life adventures?

RedBird

LESBIAN LOVE

After my cancer (lumpectomy, chemo, radiation) and the loss of my mother, I found myself full of anxiety. My resting pulse rate was 105—couldn't bring it down. I have no desire whatsoever for sex. I don't know which medication is causing it, but I could really care less. However, my partner cares tremendously; to her it is real important. I believe she has a right to want more intimacy. My partner and I were not together through my cancer, but have been since the end of my treatment. She is great in every way, and as important as this is to her, I just have no interest. I am not opposed to counseling; I have been a recovering alcoholic for almost 23 years, and have had my fair share. Just not sure what that could possibly do to influence my desires, but I will keep plugging along.

Autumn

I have experienced fear and anxiety about exposing myself in an intimate way. I have had four breast operations—two lumpectomies, one biopsy, and one partial mastectomy. My breasts do not look the same as they did but I can't begin to tell you how grateful I am to still have them. I refer to them as "my girls."

I have not been with a partner in about ten years. Decided that I needed to work on myself and that I would wait until and if the right person came into my life. Well, that happened this past September. I was visiting in Oregon and found her. Yes, I am a lesbian. I live 2,500 miles across the country so as you can imagine this is quite the courtship. I had fears about my scars, etc., but believe they tell stories and should be shared with the one I love. As a way to be supportive she has been attending a lesbian breast cancer support group. She just told me about it recently. I was touched that she wanted to be part of that part of me. So far we have not been intimate so that is a *yet.* I think the slowness and deliberate way we have gotten closer has really helped me to feel safe and cared for.

My advice is to listen to that scared voice inside that will guide you. Take it easy and be kind to yourself. Embrace the fear and know that it is all part of the process we go through to heal.

Greatful2b

SEX

Only three little letters, yet they comprise an alphabet of delight, desire, hope, misunderstanding, and confusion.

> "I can get an orgasm with batteries. For lovin', I need a partner."
>
> lambda77

My husband, the most wonderful man in the world (honestly), has not touched my unreconstructed chest wall unless I have held his hand to do it. He won't talk about why not. I can guess. He was just recovering from a significant health issue when I was diagnosed, so although sex had been great prior it's slim to none. I used to teach sexual therapy for spinal cord injured patients, so I know quite a few tricks. Sex toys help, and really nice lubricating creams are now available. But it's become the elephant in the room. It's there, it's big, but no one has the energy to deal with it!

LynneM

> "I really miss sex and wish oh I wish they could come up with an alternative for us vivacious young women."
>
> annemac

My sex drive has always been a lot higher than my husband's. He didn't understand my need for a "last time" with my breast as a "normal" woman or how I needed that physical acceptance via intimacy of my new body.

bradleyteach

My husband is 8 years younger than me. Sex was always a major component in our life. However since the menopause hit, I have become the best actress in town.

LaurieV

I think it is unrealistic for women "of a certain age" to expect the horny thrills of young sex; it was wonderful then and this is fine now; there's romance, warmth, fun, and all the sex-help products we can get.

betty

When I came down with breast cancer I went from 134 to 240 and I have not been able to lose weight with diet pills, diets, or anything; I stay the same no matter what and it seems to have totally killed my sex drive. My husband is wonderful and goes, "I just have more to love and I am beautiful," but lordy, what can I say? It worries me daily.

Now we are waiting on a test to come in on prostate cancer on him and now he is doubly scared thinking I will be looking for someone else. Why can't men ever understand sex isn't everything in a relationship. If only they would hold us, kiss us and tell us they love us without it having to lead to sex every time. Yeah, sex is fine but there are other things in life.

realtylady1

There have been many times I wished my husband would caress my surgery site but he won't touch it. It's ironic how I chase my husband around for sex now as he used to always initiate sexual contact first.

1Faith

Until my bilateral mastectomy I didn't have any trouble with my sex drive, etc. Since then, however, it's been a little different. But the other problem is that, for me, my nipples played a big part in my enjoyment of our intimacy. And I really do miss that. Yes, I can still get pleasure; it's just not as easy and takes longer. Of course my husband doesn't have any problem with *that* part. He'll take as long as I need.

little jumper

Try feeling sexy when you are 8 months pregnant with no hair.

LukesMom

I'm all for the sex toys and therapists if they'll help. I actually hosted a sex toys party last year and couldn't believe that everyone bought something!

If I remember correctly (there's that memory thing) in the beginning our sex life after chemo was laborious at best. I was in pain and my husband was trying not to hurt me. Another thing I remember from chemo is that during the really painful stage, climaxing was the best pain reliever I could find. Careful though, it is habit forming :).

hotflash

What a subject. We can all talk about breast cancer openly to everyone now but sex still seems to be something that we don't really want to talk about with our doctors. It's not just sex, it's our whole relationships that have changed. Replens is a great estrogen-free lubricant. Talking to your man and letting him know how much you still want him even though it's a little painful in the beginning helps a lot too. You have to be honest with him. You can even play with small sex toys and you would be surprised how you feel after a few months. You can do it alone but it can really turn on some men. Oral sex is also fun. Have patience but don't give up on sex. It brings great joy into any relationship even if all you can do now is cuddle.

Eve

I am not sure what to say about this just yet, because in my years on this planet I have yet to have sexual intercourse with a man (or woman for that matter). But now I am in this new relationship and my new beau of 8 months called it off last week because he has a "high libido" that was suffering (or whatever you call it). Which I knew and was working around to having such fun. Now I am ready. Today is his birthday and I would love to just get the first time over with to see what all the fuss is about. I will tell you I have found pap smears to be truly (no, really, *truly*) traumatic. So I am guessing the first few stages will be messy, uncomfortable, if not downright painful.

Picassa

I had a double mastectomy after my second bout of DCIS in the same breast. I chose no reconstruction and still have feeling in my chest wall. Our sex life is better than ever and I have had no problems with menopause. No hot flashes, no dryness in the vagina, etc. I feel so lucky after reading all the problems other women have had.

Kay

I am 5 years out and I promise things do get better.

DawnMarie

Fear of infection (or is it fear of intimacy?)

I have to admit, though not willingly, sexual intimacy has not been the highest priority on my list for the past month. Too many other thoughts whirling around in my brain. Now as we settle into the routine of treatment, I am beginning to think about it more. I get warnings about staying away from possible sources of infection. I am sure many of you have heard all of this before. Did you worry about UTI, yeast infections, lack of lubrication? Did your significant others worry about hurting you, like pressing on the port or holding you too tight and hurting the surgical site? All issues have been raised at our house. Are we just afraid of intimacy right now or do we really just have too much else to think about right now?

Scottie

My husband and I have had communication issues for years, although he would never admit it. I tried to emphasize that I needed a lubricant or I couldn't have sex. His response was pretty much "just let me get you revved up, baby (wink, wink)" or "I hate that yucky stuff!" It didn't bother him that I would end up with a bladder infection every time we had sex!

He found the hairlessness exciting and didn't mind the temporary booblessness or permanent weight gain. And though he says he's not a boob man, he loves his *Playboy* and thinks Hooters is a great family restaurant. My problem is his insensitivity to what I feel. No amount of talking has managed to get through, so after many years of trying,

I've stopped having intercourse with him. I satisfy him other ways but cringe every time he leers at me. I think I was feeling a bit used, and still am.

lambda77

INTIMACY

Because of the numerous side effects from tamoxifen, having sex has been sad, painful, and also very funny. My husband has vision problems and to see him with two pairs of readers and a little flashlight and me with two or three creams, trying to decide which combo to use, and then the two of us figuring out the next steps . . . at least we could laugh.

I thought I knew my spouse but now I know him on a deeper level. He looks at me and says I'm beautiful. I am beautiful to him, even when I don't feel attractive to myself. Sad, but when my husband was severely injured a few years ago in a car accident, he had a terrible time receiving help from me. Now I think he has actually changed through my having breast cancer and maybe can let me help him too.

Rachel

I lost both of my breasts to a bilateral mastectomy a month before my 31st birthday. I have three middle-aged children, and have been re-married to a wonderful man for the past 5 years. It's seven months post-surgery, and I enjoy the freedom of not having breasts. I have found that it doesn't make me feel like less of a woman, or less attractive when I am in public. And at home, I am very comfortable exposing my scarred chest to my husband when we are alone. I often joke about my flat chest, and feel no compulsion to wear a prosthesis. But when we are sexually intimate the depth of the loss is truly felt, and many times afterwards, I cry. I find myself reaching up to grab my breasts, and realizing they're no longer there. It is a very empty and lonely feeling. I have noticed that my husband never touches my chest anymore. We have talked about it, and I have told him that it might help me deal with some of the loss if he were to tenderly touch my scars. But I don't think he really thinks about it; out of sight, out of mind kind of thing?

But in terms of our emotional intimacy, it has deepened even beyond the sexual encounter. My husband was the one measuring the fluids and draining the drains when I came home after my surgery. My husband was the one packing my wound when an infection left a large cavity in my chest. My husband was the one decorating my bald head with henna when my hair fell out. He was the one holding my chemo pump as I showered, and helping me get dressed when I couldn't do it by myself. He painted my toenails. He shaved my legs for me. And he holds me when I cry after our times of sexual intimacy. My husband would lie in bed next to me at night and lay hands on my cancerous body as he prayed for my healing. And that is an intimacy that indeed supersedes sexual intimacy. So I would say that intimacy has deepened, and being able to freely cry over the loss of my breasts has only benefited that.

highaim

I have no trouble with sexual intimacy. My husband and I are as sexually active as we can be. The fact that we have less sex than when we first got together has more to do with the fact that my husband had a liver transplant 4 years ago than it does with my breast cancer. I used to think intimacy only meant sex but since I was diagnosed and treated for breast cancer my understanding of the word has changed. When I first got sober someone told me that "intimacy" means "into me see." My need for intimacy has definitely changed as a result of breast cancer. Today it means spending time with my loved ones and doing things for each other. I will bake a cake or type my husband's homework just because I want to. We can sit together and just laugh at the silliest stuff. I think I was too busy too often prior to breast cancer and now I have slowed down and started to look around me at all the wonderful things in my life. I am finally taking time to show my husband, his children and grandchildren, my sister and my friends how much they really mean to me and how glad I am to have them in my life. That is the true meaning of intimacy to me.

Lisabe

What I found interesting was that the day the doctor called me and told me that the tumor was cancerous, I got to experience my most intimate moment with a male friend of mine and it didn't involve sex. Intimacy holds a whole new meaning for me.

Truly Blessed

I don't think that true intimacy has anything to do with sex. I think it's a bonding of the hearts and souls. Sex can come and go but once you have found that someone you can really relate to, that can never be lost and it doesn't have to be a partner—it can be anyone.

zoochild

I've *always* been worried about being lovable and scared to be in love; breast cancer didn't change that a bit! If anything, I want an intimate relationship more than ever, because I'm aware of how short life is.

AnneMarie

I'm scared to get intimate with anyone because I fear they will freak out when they see my breast and I am afraid I will disappoint them sexually. But I sure do get awfully lonely sometimes. But I always seem to bounce back and remember that I don't need a man to be happy, and that my happiness is dependant on me and me alone! There are worse fates in life than just being alone.

justadame

YOUR VAGINA — FORGIVING AND NOT SO FORGIVING

No beating about the bush here: the women tell it like it is. Moreover, they're practically evangelical in their enthusiasm for sharing remedies to get back your mojo.

> "I feel sexy, but I'm afraid to have sex!"
>
> gloami

Lordy Lordy . . . No Drive . . . Pain . . . Dryness . . . yup, yup, yup. Chemo/chemopause, and who knows what other reasons are why I am like I am now. I am very, very fortunate to have the most supportive, patient hubby through all of this. We have made 2 agreements:

1. No quickie love making.
2. KY jelly and a product that is like natural moisture are *essential*.

I must admit though, I do feel like I am a virgin again, which amusingly enough makes hubby feel pretty darn good.

Dragonfli

> "Your vagina is a very forgiving organ."
>
> abrenner

The "no drive/pain/and dryness" are issues for me. I attribute it to lack of estrogen. If it weren't for the use of a dilator I would be dried up. My gynecologist tried to get me to go to the sex shop but I didn't have the courage.

Noel

I experienced so many intimacy issues. Initially after surgery, a lumpectomy, and re-excision I was left with very little breast tissue. I was quite small to begin with! That made me feel less desirable. The chemo didn't help. Between tiredness and vaginal dryness, intercourse became unpleasant and at times painful for me.

It has been 3 years since chemo ended; however, being on the tamoxifen for several years has resulted in severe atrophy of the vagina. A "dead" vagina at 43. Nice! This left me with a good deal of discomfort not only during sex, but also simply walking, sitting. It almost felt like little cuts and a good deal of irritation.

Good news! Several months ago my oncologist prescribed an Estring. It is a ring you insert in the vagina for 90 days at a time. It releases a very low localized dose of estrogen. Being on tamoxifen he was comfortable with me using it. It has helped greatly. Things are not "as they were" down there, but day to day is much more comfortable. Sex has become much easier too.

Elise

I too have lost my libido and the ability to have an orgasm. My oncologist also prescribed Estring, which does help quite a bit with the pain and the frequent UTIs. My husband has been very understanding but feels bad that he can no longer satisfy me. I keep telling him that it is not his fault, it is all mine. I feel bad for him because I know sexual relations are healthy for him and our relationship. But I no longer cringe at the thought of the pain since the Estring.

Rosie Posey

You are going to laugh out loud when you read this, but it really works! In addition to using lubricants you should buy the smallest "dose" of vitamin E. Starting with maybe twice a week when you go to bed, insert this vitamin E in your vagina! Yes, you read it correctly. After a while cut down to once a week and eventually probably less. My gynecologist told me to do this and she says it really helps; she can tell during her exams that the lining of my vagina is in good shape. Gives new meaning to taking your vitamin E, doesn't it?!

WalkinBoobs

"A 'dead' vagina at 43. Nice!"

Elise

Okay, I'm going to share something very few people know about me. I have a condition that causes me to clench up at the vaginal opening whenever anything (tampon, finger, speculum, penis) is inserted. It makes penetration *very* painful if left untreated, or if I go a long time without sex. It's a physical manifestation of psychological trauma. (I'd had a couple of rough experiences by the time I was 21—not abuse.)

Anyway, when I was 22 I started with the gynecologist I still see. She had a difficult time examining me for many years. I would be *so* humiliated and embarrassed. She said something to me back then that she still giggles over today when I remind her. But it's really true. She told me, "The vagina is a very forgiving organ."

In other words, as one of you put it so well, "use it or lose it." She taught me exercises to self-dilate, she's had me use Replens and Astroglide (insufficient lubrication really *does* affect pain and insertion issues), and I've had a *lot* of counseling, yoga, visualization, and meditation to help me learn to breathe and relax through the clench.

My point is, you really *can* bring your body back to functional status. And from experience I can tell you that you can find your way back to pleasure as well. It won't be the same, but it will still be nice. Really nice. Good luck. Take your time. Enjoy the process as much as you can. Share the ride with your partner if you can. Relax. Breathe. Your vagina is a very forgiving organ.

abrenner

I had cancer when I was 39. The chemo put me into menopause for good. I also had an oophorectomy [surgical removal of one or both ovaries]. I do remember how I lost my drive. I also had small kids at the time. No one talked about vaginal dryness and losing your sex drive. Why can't doctors tell you this? I suppose that they give you enough bad news. They don't want to tell you everything. It was really tough. I remember someone telling me about Astroglide for the dryness (a guy must have invented it to name it that), but it worked and I did get more of a drive back when I wasn't so tired.

sunny

MASTURBATION

The bottom line here is that for you or your spouse, it's a win-win situation, perhaps even a healing one.

I want to address the masturbation issue, though, since many people feel uncomfortable discussing this and perhaps this "anonymous" site is the best forum for this. For those of you who have not tried before, it really does help keep you feeling good and also more physically flexible. Some of you may have religious/upbringing/other reasons for not wanting to try, but it is not harmful and I believe it is a healthy part of taking care of yourself, especially if you don't have a partner or it's too much pain/stress to be intimate with a man right now. Dare to try it. You may be surprised, and you certainly won't hurt anyone.

songbird

This is a sensitive subject and I think at times my husband has tried the same during the nights but I do not know for sure. It hurts me the most that I cannot be there for him as I used to. How can I lie next to this wonderful man and not please him, or me for that matter. The thought of him after being married to me for over 21 years having to take matters in his own hands brings tears to my eyes and would be the one thing I would like to change if I could since all of my diagnosis, treatment, and recovery.

See, I am not selfish in that I would not change the fact that I have this disease but to please my husband would be the greatest gift of all. So I wait for the medical community to come to address this issue for women that have far too many other things to deal with than to not complete their wants and desires and vows as a woman and wife.

Mel

Mel, thanks for sharing your feelings so expressively. I agree that it is not a matter of being selfish or not, but of course we want to share all forms of love with our partners, especially those who have stood by us in the darkest days, and I want my husband to be happy and fulfilled also. I hope, with you, that better solutions to this dilemma will be found, for all of us. In the meantime, we do our best.

songbird

YOUR LIBIDO: JUST LIKE THE MOON, IT WAXES, IT WANES, IT EVEN COMES BACK AGAIN

> "I want a syrupy thick bottle of desire!"
>
> Stormy

I find that my bigger problem is no libido. I mean no interest at all!! I am in my second marriage and was quite the horny devil when we united. Now I'm like a dud.

Raesinthesun

> "Sex is not painful or unpleasant, just not interesting."
>
> SarahBF

Estrogen depletion with estrogen-positive breast cancer makes for dry (grind-grind) sex and lack of interest. You can use all the glides, jellies, toys, etc., but what about the desire? I want to *feel* horny! Remember that, ladies??? I am fairly comfortable with my self-image. I have worked hard at this after being taken off tamoxifen, gotten my Masters, taking Effexor for hot flashes (love that stuff!), but I want a syrupy thick bottle of desire! My hubby goes along (what a keeper), but our 20-something marriage could use the boost with all the adolescent problems and divorce around us!

Stormy

I am so relieved to hear others voice the fact that your sex drive is in the toilet. Mine too. I was on tamoxifen (and in pseudo-menopause) for 8 years (my 1st bout was when I was 28), then my periods came back when I went off of it. Then I went through natural menopause at 39, and with my 2nd bout of breast cancer am on Arimidex. We just didn't know how much we loved that estrogen! It never dawns on me to initiate anything. My husband is sooo wonderfully understanding. He likes KY Jelly (I don't know if he really does, or just says this). I do take my shirt off (upon request only); he thinks I'm beautiful anyway. I do notice that he never touches "it" though. This makes me feel weird. I've had reconstruction, so the implants are always there between us. He is so open to trying things to make me more comfortable and I really appreciate him for this. Our love for each other was great before, but it has definitely grown stronger for having weathered breast cancer.

slr

I have not worried about being lovable; I've not been scared to be in love. At 7 months out of chemo, I have no desire to have sex. It's not that I have vaginal dryness, which I don't; I have virtually no desire. In fact, thinking about sex has brought forth feelings of revulsion.

    KeyWoman

My problem is also no libido. I feel good about myself, I am working out, lost a few pounds, and look pretty sexy for 54, but it is hard to get in the mood for sex. My husband is very understanding; he's hoping that "this too shall pass" and I will be the old me again.

    kgirl

I was frustrated at first by the loss of libido. Now I'm resigned and that's frightening. I'd like to know: would I have lost almost all desire by the age of 52 anyway? Or is it the result of the chemo and inability to take hormones since my cancer was hormone receptive?

    dhinsvark

I too suffer from loss of libido. Horrible for my husband, although I think I've been okay with it. I did find one thing that helped me. I suffer from vaginal dryness, and of course during sex that can be painful. I discovered that using Viacreme has helped me. My doctor said it is okay as it doesn't have any hormones in it, since I am ER positive. It stimulates the clitoral region (can I say that?) when applied, and has a menthol-type effect, which gets me more "in the mood." Many women use it to obtain orgasms.

    surviving soul

For years because of all my surgeries and surgical menopause I haven't wanted sex, haven't cared for it, haven't been physically up for it, and, well, my hubby is wonderful and understanding so it's been pretty lousy but worked for us. But now—oh gosh I can't believe I'm sharing this—now, believe it or not, I really crave my hubby. I mean for one, the man is soooo sexy and adorable and the love of my life. But with vaginal atrophy the vagina is so small that *nothing* fits up there anymore and there is no stimulation. Nothing works. How awfully ironic. Now I crave him and need him, with all my heart and soul, and I want to show him love in ways I haven't been able to and now I can't.

Princess86

MENOPAUSE

I am 37 years old but have been in medical menopause for 4 years. My friends are having babies and I am having hot flashes.

Kim W

> "I went into menopause two years ago and my brain went out the window."
>
> Cath

I hold my friends' babies and my insides fall to pieces because I know that I don't have the option of having more children if we wanted, between being in treatment for so long and being forced into early menopause.

cpr1964

COMMUNICATE, COMMUNICATE, COMMUNICATE

This was a really tough one for me. My husband had not approached me in a sexual way and when I would do things to encourage it, sex never seemed to be in the plans. I really was beginning to feel rejected, but at the same time he was doing so many other intimate things for me and helping out so. He is very private. When I asked him if he would like to see the scar from the modified radical mastectomy, he immediately popped out a NO! I was afraid that he did not want to see my body. It took some courage, but I asked him one night why we didn't have sex anymore. Was he afraid of hurting me? Did the idea of the scar bother him? His response: "There's nothing wrong with you! I just can't get it up!" You cannot imagine the laughter we had together when we both realized that each one was worried about the other's reaction. That conversation relieved a tremendous amount of stress for us both.

Linda

The key is communicating with your partners about why we have the low libidos, i.e., meds/menopause. Often they misunderstand and take our lack of interest as rejection. I know for me, now that I'm losing some of my menopausal weight, I feel better about myself. This was a real issue for me because my reconstruction needs some revisions which insurance won't allow because they see it as purely cosmetic. They have no idea how it effects us emotionally.

ANA

I have been with my husband for 27 years, married for 20 (!) and we always have had a good sex life, until he had a minor heart attack at age 41 (runs in his family). Since then, it has been sporadic, and although he is healthy now and I have few physical reasons other than fatigue to stop me, we usually just avoid the subject unless circumstances are perfect, which is rare with two kids, work, and everything else. For us I think it is mostly a communications issue: we have been so involved in talking about so many other important things we have just put sex on the back burner, although we love each other very much and have no intentions of ever leaving each other. I am planning to tackle the issue this summer when things slow down a little, since I think in addition to the sheer physical enjoyment, it is healthier for us to make love more often, and I think we'd feel even closer if we did. I am committed to celebrating my 20th anniversary fully, though, so this is not a dead issue for me!

songbird

My husband (of 27 years) has always been a poor communicator. He keeps everything well hidden inside himself. I too have to admit I feel sorry for him, sorry that he can't open up more and at least *try* to share some of those feelings. Unfortunately it is very difficult to break ingrained habits of stoical, Ohioan farmers, and that is the stock from which he comes. Most of his family is the same way. His own mother never interferes or even states an opinion about any of her children now, or when they were younger. I, on the other hand, am "Mrs. Butt-insky," and welcome to my club!! It consists of me asking and probing and offering opinions every chance I get! My husband has never understood that, and it actually irritates him at times, but I still do it because that's who I am, and if friends or family members don't like it, I am of the impression they would tell me, and I can't remember anyone ever telling me so!

    carolecare

The sex life just disappeared and I was so upset and so sad and didn't know how to talk to my husband about it. The women in my support group told me that it probably was that he was scared of hurting me. They told me to just be honest and talk to him about what I was feeling. So I did and he too assured me that was all it was. He didn't marry me for my hair or how much I weighed. He loved me for me and no matter what he wasn't going anywhere. He wanted me to set the tone and let him know if I was up to it or not. He knew that my body was in pain and really was petrified of hurting me. So from then on things in that aspect got back to normal. I really am blessed for having such a great friend and lover in my husband.

    sibling rivalry

" 'I AM WOMAN,' BOOBS OR NO BOOBS"

I am still the "lovable person" I was before. Only now if I want to give someone a hug, my breasts don't get in the way and I don't have to

worry about exciting someone I shouldn't. When my husband became sick my only thoughts and desires were to take care of him and
make things as comfortable as I could. I was only 41 at the time so I
was not dead to that part of me. It just didn't seem important to me;
I didn't get any hot sexual urges or anything. Just the fact that he was
there and we could hold one another was wonderful. We united in a
different way, spiritually.

After he passed on I didn't have time or energy left to even think
about sex and wasn't interested in finding another man for any reason. "I am Woman," boobs or no boobs.

NMRose

I am single and 49. A/C threw me into menopause. Has having
breast cancer changed my sex life? No! I wasn't "getting any" before
and I'm still not! Actually, though, having cancer has, very surprisingly, made me more attractive to men! I have a lot of guys interested
in me, new and old. Maybe it is the new attitude that came with the
cancer. I am much more open. I don't have any burning desire for
sex, but I am loving the attention and caring. I have been on tamoxifen
for three years. I can tell that I am all shriveled up. It would probably
hurt if I ever did become active. I also have vaginal discharge, and
rarely-occurring herpes. When I was first diagnosed, my guy friends
said they liked "me," not my breasts. My dentist, whose wife had
breast cancer, said he was glad to have his wife alive; he did not care
about the blob on her chest. Apparently, men have come a long way
since junior high. You don't need someone in your life that rejects you
because of the loss of your breast. I could care less if someone saw my
chest (mastectomy). Another attitude change from long ago.

Peony

A healthy sex life is part of life. Now the question: What will the new
man in your life think about you? My thought is this. You have just
gone through somewhat of a life/death experience. Your first question

to yourself should be: Do you want someone who is going to love you superficially (on the outside) or do you want someone to love you for who you really are? If you give the second answer, you've made the right choice. If a man really cares about who you are, he will stay. If he only cares about what you look like, then you are in for a life of misery. This is your chance to choose what really matters in life and what doesn't. Only you can make that choice, just as you did while making the choice to have a lumpectomy, treatment, and reconstruction. Please don't put the pressure on yourself of what other people (especially men) are going to think about you. There are only two opinions that count, yours and God's.

zoochild

CHAPTER EIGHT

Basic Relationships, A to Z

"What happened for me around relationships
after breast cancer was no less than a
life-changing way of dealing with people
in my life."

sawiam

*Think of all the relationships in your life: parents and chil-
dren, spouses and significant others, friends and extended
family, the dog groomer and cat sitter, coworkers and clients,
even the person who delivers your mail or does your dry cleaning. To
paraphrase the poet John Donne, no woman is an island. When I was
dealing with breast cancer, relationships with every thing and every
one changed for me; even years later the impact resonates. Some of the
friends who were especially present in my life at that time have drifted
to the periphery; others are just as central to my life. I know I'm lucky
that my best friends then are still my best friends. Yet the physical
therapist who was my lifeblood when it came to healing from surgery
is now just a name on a Rolodex card, although she remains special in
my memory. It's easy to become bitter about the people we think should
be more understanding or sympathetic, and it's lousy to endure some of*

the things people say. Of the many relationships described here, I find myself the most upset when I read some of the unthinking, unblinking things people said to the women here. Consider how you would respond to this: the husband who says of his wife after her bandages are removed, "Oh look, Bride of Frankenstein." Or what do you say when someone tells you they know of a woman who has just died from breast cancer? And what woman here hasn't been asked that withering question, "But really, how are you?" Ouch.

On the flip side is the value of your many relationships. Who matters more in your life? How have you achieved closer bonds, or had the courage to loosen less healthy ones? And what about the person on the street? Did you bring any more tolerance and understanding to strangers who crossed your path? I remember one night I was standing in line for a movie when a woman cut in and was talking obnoxiously loud. My first response was to say something to her; my "newer" response was to do nothing and instead think to myself, "Maybe this woman has had some catastrophe in her life. Maybe she's doing the best she can just by going out to see a movie. Maybe this is her on a good day." Being a bit more generous-spirited at that moment helped me feel better. And in the end, isn't that what we want from any relationship—to make others feel good, and to feel good about ourselves?

This isn't a true lexicon of relationships, but it is meant to suggest the vast array of people with whom we interact, all of them meaningful to one degree or another. Most of these are short anecdotes, sometimes covered more elaborately in other chapters of the book.

"I live a life with much more intention and presence than I ever did before and I do it through my relationships."

sawiam

"My relationship to myself has changed the most since breast cancer."

betty

COWORKERS

It was the outpouring of support that got me through my surgery. I was amazed at the number of people that dropped off dinners, sent cards and flowers. My coworkers put a basket together of wonderful, fun items for me. Lotions, cards, books, CDs, garden gloves, poker games, you name it—the basket was overflowing with items of support and love. When word got around about my having cancer, people I hadn't worked with in over 10 years were contacting me.

mamacolette

I think the worst thing anyone said to me was a coworker. She informed me that since I had breast cancer last year and got all the attention, I should let someone else get the attention this year. I really think she was jealous that everyone coming back after summer vacation was asking how I was doing. Such is life.

special kids

I remember the kindness of many strangers. I interviewed for a new job just after my hair was growing back. It was probably the first week I started going out in public without a hat. Not only did the guy hire me, I never once felt like my short, spiked, stupid-looking hair mattered to him. I didn't want my cancer to affect his decision to hire me so I did not mention it for a few months. His only response was, "I am proud to have you on my team and it would not have changed my decision."

Captiva96

FAMILY

Other than my own children, the only immediate family I have is my sister. We had never been extremely close, but after my diagnosis we began sharing a lot more. We are now best friends. Another relationship which opened up was the one between me and my ex-husband, the father of my four children. Any anger he might have harbored vanished, and we now have a wonderful, caring, best friend sort of relationship also. He probably knows me better than anyone.

scrapper

> "My sister saw a 'new side' of me when I was sick, and I'm seeing a 'new side' of my husband now. Now I'm looking for an opportunity to 'be there' for someone else. The wheel keeps turning . . ."
>
> Cath

My son was grown and recently married when I was diagnosed. He took his cue from me. If I was strong and positive, he responded in the same way. My son, daughter-in-law, and new granddaughter walk with me and my husband on Mother's Day in the Komen Race for the Cure and are active in our local ACS Relay for Life. I think a certain admiration comes with staring the beast in the face and holding your ground.

Gram K

Some of my close family members have been surprisingly distant. Even though my chemo experience has been pretty tolerable, and I'm working part time and continuing to be active, they don't seem to know what to say to me beyond "How was your last treatment?" It's been disappointing that some of the people who know me best now see me only as a cancer patient.

Towanda2

My mama was devastated. My sister had to go be with my mama and calm her down. We live four hours apart. When I had my surgery, my mama, sister, brother, husband, son, daughter-in-law, my best friend, and my boss were there. I think the nurses were a little disturbed because I had so many people in the recovery room. My youngest son was scared to come to the hospital. He didn't come to see me for a couple of days after. He couldn't stand to see me like that. But once he did, he felt better because I was doing so good.

DollyD

FRIENDSHIPS

When I was diagnosed, I was recently divorced with three teenagers and no family nearby. I have four friends who pitched in and took care of me. My chemo treatments were every third Friday, so on the night before chemo, we would go out to a restaurant and party. Everyone in the restaurant always knew we were the chemo team out for dinner before chemo. I think I am the only chemo patient that ever went into treatment with a hangover.

One of these friends also took pictures of each dinner and the chemo nurses and doctors so now I have a lovely album with many fond memories to go along with the negative side of the whole ordeal. Another friend arrived on the day I was being discharged with a beautifully wrapped present. To my amazement, she had made me a beautiful quilt. She explained that when she would leave the hospital at night, she was too wound up to sleep, so she sewed me her very first quilt. I sleep with it every night still, nearly 3 years later. Funny, a 50-year-old woman with a security blanket.

shelleyk

I had a childhood friend with whom I had lost touch with and through this disease, we reconnected. She, too, is a cancer survivor. She sent me a package full of scarves to brighten up my days. I loved the fact that I could write her and ask her questions and she was always there to calm me, hug me—virtually—and reassure me that I would get through whatever was going on. Talking to someone who I *knew* and went through what I was going through was truly a comfort.

Jacquie

I have a friend who means well, but constantly refers to my having had breast cancer. If we're talking about depression, aches and pains, other medical problems she always says, "You had to face and deal with breast cancer. You're a survivor." I don't mind telling people about my breast cancer, but I don't like hearing about it over and over. I feel that I dealt with it pretty well from the beginning, and don't need someone to remind me of it all the time.

Linque

I remember when I was first diagnosed and folks wanted to hook me up with other breast cancer survivors. Whenever anyone mentioned someone who had had a mastectomy I thought: "Why do they want me to talk with her? I'm not having a mastectomy!" So, one mastectomy later, I realize that the lines we draw once diagnosed are just as fragile (and false) as the lines we draw before diagnosis. Women who've never had breast cancer are afraid of what we've had because they know it might happen to them just as easily, just as we're afraid of what might still happen to us. Recovery is a process that goes on for life.

oceanwalker

I lost my *best friend* two weeks after surgery. I sensed there was a problem when she didn't even call to see if I made it through surgery. She couldn't handle the "stress" of having a friend with cancer! Imagine my stress! The good news is that people who I considered casual friends came out of the woodwork to be supportive, etc. I have gained some very close "new" friends to take her place!

Doreen

Since most of my friends are senior citizens, there is a great empathy for our health status. But the bottom line is that at the end of our conversations we tell each other how much we love each other and that we appreciate each day and we take one minute at a time and make time to find something to smile about each day. We also e-mail each other jokes all the time—I have a collection of such e-mails that keep me smiling.

en share-a-smile

She was diagnosed at the age of 74.

I was particularly concerned about how one of my friends would take my diagnosis. He is a gay male hairdresser—very handsome and conscious of appearance in dress and looks. (He could be one of the Fab Five on *Queer Eye*.) I also knew he was positively phobic about cancer, refusing even to say the word. But he and I have known each other since we were in our high school band together. Now, middle-aged and sharing a pew in the same church, I wondered how he would respond to my diagnosis.

When the last of my hair fell out and I showed up at church the first time in a wig I had picked out of the American Cancer catalogue, he seemed not to notice my new look. The next Sunday, he handed me a small gift bag and said, "This is for you. I think you'll like it, but wait until you get home to open the bag." At home, later in the day, I opened the bag to find a beautiful wig, the perfect size, shape, and color with a super soft lining to protect my tender scalp. The wig looked so astonishingly like my own hair that, when I wore it, other friends were puzzled and thought perhaps I hadn't lost my hair after all.

The next time I saw him, I had on "his" wig. We laughed, hugged, and talked. He was able to stand his ground in the face of "cancer talk" and even told me he had searched for the softest wig base he could find to protect my bare scalp. I think he felt empowered and proud of himself for not running. The memory of his kindness, his gift, and his desire to deal with his cancer phobia for my sake remains one of the morale-boosting touchstones in my life with cancer. Here's to friends who stay!! They are the salt of the earth!!

mountainmomma

I had great support from friends, one of whom even cut her hair very short in support of my hair loss! Some were a little too directive, telling me what I should do or feel. And some would call me to console them when their life wasn't going well, but for the most part, my friends were a terrific source of encouragement and support. Along the way, I've let go of some who were draining me emotionally, all take and no give. Those few relationships were ones I should have ended long before, and breast cancer just helped open my eyes to these one-way relationships.

nonnazano

My favorite response to news of breast cancer? One friend e-mailed me back: "That f***ing sucks!" No pussy-footing, no "it couldn't have happened to a better person" or "you're so young!" Just the bald, visceral truth of it. It sucks!

MCN

During the middle of my chemo a girlfriend was trying to get me out of the house and I finally agreed to go. We were sitting in a booth having coffee at a local restaurant and a table full of older men was near us and while we were talking an older man looked over at us and smarted off: "Women will do anything to get attention. I just don't know why her hairdresser would ever do anything so crazy." The lady I was with raised up real slow. I said, "No, don't say anything," and the next thing I knew this 98-pound when-she-was-wet lady had raised the man up by his collar and said, "I want you to apologize to her right now, she has cancer," and the man's face went white. He was muttering, "I didn't know." He said, "Lady, I am really sorry. You see so much stuff nowadays I thought you were just experimenting with something new." Needless to say I didn't go with her to a café till my hair came back. But you couldn't ask for a better friend.

realtylady1

GENERAL

> "We take each other for granted less and say 'I love you' more."
>
> Lizzi

One of the biggest lessons I've learned so far has come from the wide variety of responses from family, friends, and coworkers. I've never been close to anyone with cancer or any serious illness and previously had no idea what to say or do when I heard about someone who was recovering from surgery or undergoing treatment.

Following my surgery I received many, many cards wishing me well. I could never have imagined how important such a small, simple gesture would be. It didn't matter whether the sender wrote a personal message or simply "thinking of you." Just to know that all these people cared about me was a tremendous boost to my spirits.

Towanda2

> "Kindness begins at home."
>
> songbird

Having breast cancer changed all my relationships in some way or other. My daughter, who is 32 and has a daughter of her own, became very anxious about possibly losing me and also about developing breast cancer herself. We talked and cried a lot about it at first. It made us closer, in part because we take each other for granted less. My son, 34, is mostly unable to talk about my cancer. He can deal with it in small bits, but the idea of it can be too much. Sometimes I need to talk about it with him, and he tries to listen and asks for information, or about my feelings, but then he'll change the subject. I feel lonely and separated from him when this happens. My two stepsons are another part of the story. We have been family for many years, but I have never been sure they really accepted me. When they learned of my cancer they really stepped up, and expressed a lot of interest and concern. I was pleasantly surprised. My mother-in-law is more like a mother to me than my own mother, and she cried with me when I first told her.

All these relationships, as well as several others, have become more intense and precious because we have been reminded that you never know what will happen and how long you will have each other. We take each other for granted less and say "I love you" more.

Lizzi

What happened for me around relationships after breast cancer was no less than a life-changing way of dealing with people in my life. After breast cancer it seemed that I was unable to deal with any relationship that was close and personal unless it was real. It was like the experience of those 3 to 4 months of coming through the fire let me see very clearly that relationships are the most important thing in life and I just couldn't tolerate those that were not nurturing to me.

I also really learned what I want and need out of friendships and love and what I don't. In this way my experience has been invaluable.

I live a life with much more intention and presence than I ever did before and I do it through my relationships.

sawiam

My relationship to myself has changed the most since breast cancer. I do feel proud that I am able to continue my life with two breast cancers—definitely stronger. I sort of surprised myself. I did not include my college sons too much in my treatments and illness; they are aware of it all but see me as fine and that's the way I like it. As for friends, they are all still there although the few people I really did not like but tolerated are gone—I don't have time for them. What a relief that was!

betty

I think that my parents are very special people. They would like to see me retire from teaching just because they think it would be better for my health. If I need something, all I have to do is tell them, and they will make sure that it gets done. My whole family is that way. Cancer has done nothing but make us closer if that was possible.

My relationships with my husband and family and friends and coworkers grew stronger, and I learned that my relationship with my community was also strong. I guess that was the surprise. I didn't know so many people cared about me until cancer hit.

Linda

I found that talking about what I was going through helped me, whether anyone else appreciated it or not. I actually would look for other women in stores without hair and eyebrows, just to maybe get the chance to talk to them.

Cancer does some strange things to folks; I think it brings out all the insecurities that have been there all along, and gives them an excuse to surface and make themselves known. Go ahead: feel bad, get mad, scream, get real good and angry but make sure you direct your anger at the cause—cancer—and not the person.

jennagram

One of my best friends, who also took care of my kids while I worked, left me a single pink rose every time I had a chemo treatment. (She had a house key.) She and another friend shaved my head while we sipped champagne when most of my hair had fallen out!

I think friends were the most supportive because the emotions that they have during the situation are different than those of family. And sometimes family members get caught up in doing or saying the right thing.

junebug

I think family members and close friends don't know *what* to say so they avoid us. I think we have to be the brave ones and call them and start talking about what we would usually talk about—the kids, grandkids, baseball, whatever you would have talked to them about before. We have to let them know that we are still *us*, and that cancer doesn't define us.

Nett

I have found that most people are very unknowledgeable when it comes to the subject of cancer. I was through surgery and in chemo when I really started to notice that the majority of people I had always been around were no longer coming over or even calling. The turning point was when my significant other and I were invited to one of his friends' for a party. I was given a paper cup, plate, and plastic silverware, while everyone else was using regular glasses, plates, and silverware. They actually thought they could catch "it" from me. Needless to say, I didn't stay long and was very hurt.

siggy001

It is surprising who really comes through and who may mean to but just can't for whatever reason. I have solidified some old friendships, let some slide, and made some great new friends, all through this experience. My family has drawn closer, as have my oldest friends from school days. My husband and I have worked through some communications issues that we had building up before both of us got sick, and I think although we will always have to be vigilant (both being the "suffer in silence" types), cancer has made our relationship stronger overall. As to my relationship with myself, well, I am trying to be more forgiving of my faults and less demanding of others, and I am trying to "hear" myself better than I used to with all the rushing around. I feel mostly strong, but also able to be fragile when I need to, without judging myself too harshly. Kindness begins at home.

 songbird

GOD

I have become a lot closer to God. I know my spirit, my faith, has grown and now I take time no matter what to thank God personally for each blessing He has given me. I believe He has given me a cure, through all the prayers that were said for me. So if anything, this cancer has opened my eyes to all the wonderful people I have in my life and the greatness of God to have the medical field so vigorously trying to find a cure for cancer!

 lilybelle2

Two things I heard a lot, which drove me crazy.

 1: "Bet you're mad at God for this, huh?!"
  Nope, never blamed God or thought I deserved this. To which I
  consistently heard, "Well, you're just in denial."
 2: "God never gives us more than we can handle."

I felt like having a T-shirt made with that phrase and my footnote, "I just wish he didn't trust me so much!"

Janet

HUSBANDS

What do you say when all of a sudden "till death do us part" seems closer than you *ever* anticipated?

Princess86

The night of my lumpectomy my husband slept in my room at the hospital. I can't tell you how important that was, looking over from my bed and seeing him there all night. It made the fear manageable.

Lizzi

My husband of 33 years and I have gotten much closer since my diagnosis. The night before each treatment he'll call me at work and ask "May I take you out for dinner tonight?"

Towanda2

I think my relationships didn't change but my perception of them did. I have a very outgoing husband and sometimes feel a little in his shadow with our couple friends. When I was diagnosed, the outpouring of love and concern surprised me. I finally realized they cared about me for me, not just that I'm married to a great guy.

ritavv

I saw a totally different side of my husband during my breast cancer. I am so appreciative of his support and encouragement. I have told many people that I could never have made it through the cancer without him. The first day of my chemo, as we are sitting there together waiting, he took my hand and said he wished he could do this for me.

brinda

My husband survived a liver transplant 4 years ago. He was sick for two years before the transplant so when I was diagnosed he just looked at it like it was his turn to take care of me. We have an additional bond that can't be broken.

Lisabe

MOTHERS

I think that my relationship with my mother has turned a corner since I had breast cancer. My mom lives in another state and was not able to come to be with me during and after my surgery. I think that my illness hit her really hard—her oldest child having a possibly fatal illness. I did notice that my mom called me a lot more and said that she loved me a lot more during my therapies and recovery. Since then she has had an abnormal mammogram and a biopsy that was negative. She said that she appreciates how strong I was to go through everything that I did since just the little bit that she had to go through with her biopsy was very traumatic for her. I think that she admires me for what I have been through and that I am a role model for herself, my sisters and their daughters.

Suzette

> "My mother used to say, 'When people ask how you feel, tell them you're fine, because they really don't want to hear your problems.' This applies to the curiosity seekers, not the very dearest."
>
> Linque

My mother was diagnosed a year after me. We didn't have any idea that breast cancer would be lurking in our futures. I had chemo and radiation, she had radiation. I am into the web sites and information and my mom would rather not know. I tell her anyway. We managed.

We walked in the Komen walks together in our brightly colored pink T-shirts and also in the Relay for Life walks.

DianaRmn

When I told my mother (long distance, on the phone) that I had breast cancer, she said, "Oh no, what will I do without you?"

I have never questioned how much my mother loves me, and I still don't. Several times at very low points in my life, she has said similarly insensitive things. I think the reason they leave me standing with my mouth gaping open is because even though I am the only cherished daughter, when the chips are really down, her immediate thoughts are so unfeeling and selfish.

San

When I came home for treatment, I stayed with my mother for 7 months. She was nurturing, supportive and incredibly practical, helping me figure out finances, scheduling, and taking notes at the doctors' when I was fuzzy from chemo brain.

My frustration is not with her but for her. Many of her friends abandoned her during this time, including one who my mother had supported during two bouts of breast cancer that she had had (the friend, not my mother). I think it's vital that support people get support themselves and, as the cancer patient, it wasn't something I could do for her.

MCN

PETS: ANOTHER NAME FOR FUR BABIES

"Most people think of pets as dumb animals but I have to question who the dumb one is."

zoochild

I had never thought too deeply about this and probably have taken it for granted, but my parrots and dog were the calm during the storm for me. In fact, one of my umbrella cockatoos, Angel, who is normally the devil's spawn, was by my side almost all the time. The day I got diagnosed, I came home and lay down on the bed. When I'm home she (and the other cockatoo) are allowed out of their cages. That day, Angel climbed on the bed, stood on my chest and clear as a bell said, "I love you." That was only the second time she's ever said that to me.

Then came the day I had my first chemo treatment. The anti-nausea meds gave me a horrible sinus headache. When I got home, I laid down on the couch, with a cool cloth over my forehead. Again, Angel climbed up and stood on my chest, looked me in the eye and asked, "You all right?" She's always near me when I'm home, and if I dare to put on a pair of shoes, she attacks those instead. This girl is smart: she knows shoes take me away.

KeyWoman

> "All animals give us unconditional love and I wish you all could know the peace of sitting on a hillside on a glorious afternoon with your dog at your side. It's as though I am already in heaven."
>
> Eve

My dog was my cancer buddy. He was just a puppy. We got him in April and I was diagnosed in July. When I came home after my chemo I would just lay in the bed for two days. That little guy lay right next to me, and any time I got up he would be there to lick my face or snuggle with me. I preferred to go to chemo alone and I didn't want to drag anyone else into my suffering. I did it to protect myself. I didn't want to face their faces or questions. But that little dog never had a question or a sad face. All he had was love.

My husband yells at me, but I still let the dog on the bed. It is his reward for taking such good care of me during chemo.

MJ

It has been proven that those of us who have pets (fur babies) lead a longer more peaceful life. Having said that, I would like to introduce you to my Gaby. Gaby came home to me on a Sunday screaming her little lungs out. My then neighbor brought her home from church to me. I had just lost my former cat to anaphylactic shock five days earlier. Gaby was maybe four weeks old and weighed maybe 20 ounces. (She had been abandoned by her biological mom.) It was an instant bond. I was now her mommy.

The saying that dogs have owners, cats have staff is very appropriate. We often think that cats don't listen but they do, they just choose not to respond. My Gaby responds at least 95 percent of the time. She is a great teacher and companion. Any time I feel like giving up, I just remind myself how hard she fought to stay alive in those first couple of weeks. She has the spirit of a lioness and the temperament of a clown.

zoochild

I too have a "fur baby," as you call them (great name). Mine came to me the day before my last chemo. Mylo (short for "my love") was the best thing that came out of the whole experience. I wouldn't trade him for the best looking, wealthiest single man in all of New England.

Truly Blessed

Animals absolutely know when something is wrong. They have that innate sense about them. Did you know that they have trained dogs to specifically sniff out cancer in people? I saw a documentary on that a few years ago. Most people think of pets as dumb animals but I have to question who the dumb one is.

zoochild

SISTERS: BIOLOGICAL SISTERS, BREAST CANCER SISTERS, AND SISTERS-IN-LAW

My only blood sister and I drew especially close because right after my diagnosis she had her first mammogram. They found microscopic precancerous calcifications that they removed in a simple office procedure. That one incident helped me make it through my treatments with the knowledge that my breast cancer could very possibly have prevented my sister from having to go through it.

Lisabe

I don't feel as comfortable discussing my fears about recurrence and the future with my healthy friends as I do my friends with breast cancer. My breast cancer sisters know what I am talking about because they are feeling it too. It is difficult to communicate that once you have breast cancer, or any cancer for that matter, your perspective about the future is quite different. So I have learned how much to share with healthy friends and open up much differently with my breast cancer sisters.

Raesinthesun

There are many people who don't know what to say and haven't yet learned that it's best to say nothing. I was more bothered with the sad look and pity in the tone of voice. While working through the first bout, none of my customers were aware until at least a year later. I always kept a positive attitude at work and my wig was almost a perfect match to my hair color and style. I think the fact that not many people knew kept me from listening to the pity and feeling sorry for myself. Once I was back on my feet, a small sisterhood was formed with other breast cancer patients.

tuppie

Being a small breasted woman anyway (and my then husband didn't mind a bit!), my sisters-in-law used to joke about my, ahem, stature. I got used to the jokes and took them in stride for a lot of years. After the mastectomy, one sister-in-law still thought it necessary to chime in with "Well, I can't tell which one she had cut off!" (They all talk in the third person as if you are not there.) Stupid? Oh yeah! Of course, we don't talk much because of my marriage breaking up, so along with a great husband, I lost a mouthy sister-in-law! Sometimes things just work out for the better!

Ladyblue930

> "My breast cancer sisters know what I am talking about because they are feeling it too."
>
> Raesinthesun

Things People Say . . .

hen children say some-thing that's on the cusp of good manners or slightly loopy, we think it's cute. When adults do, we're understandably less tolerant.

People say weird things and tell me stories of someone they knew who died; it makes me wonder what motivates them. I stay away from talking about it with certain people if they do this. I can understand that most people who haven't had a cancer diagnosis wouldn't know what to say, but some of the remarks are just dumb.

teddygirl

"Cancer does some strange things to folks; I think it brings out all the insecurities that have been there all along, and gives them an excuse to surface and make themselves known."

−jennagram

"It drove my husband crazy when people told him our cancer journey would make us stronger. We were fine being weak!"

−mtn woman

I hated when I was on treatment and somebody would tell me "a relative had breast cancer and died." I got to the point where I would say "If it doesn't have a good ending I don't want to know."

dreamer

I get sick of hearing what a blessing cancer should be. I have had many blessings in my life up to this point. Please don't get me wrong, I have all the faith in the Lord, but I could have done without this blessing.

DollyD

I went to a meeting and the speaker started with "the ones that found the blessing when they were diagnosed with cancer." I asked if she had cancer, she told me no. Well, I really told her the reality of what cancer patients have to go through—and then left the meeting.

dreamer

Another pet hate is someone saying that they know exactly how I feel. They don't, they can't, so why pretend.

kimbasa

The hardest comment to hear repeatedly was, "It's only hair; it'll grow back." I never said it out loud, but my first reaction was, "Yeah, but it's not YOUR @##%&* hair, is it?!?!" It's one thing to feel like shit; it's quite another to have to look like it, too.

After a while, I realized that people want so much to say something. Some do say the wrong thing, but it's not intentional. I think it's worse when people say nothing at all; that's very hard to take. It accentuates one's feelings of isolation.

metsfan

> "I think by living our normal lives and being out in the community we are examples to people that you can get cancer, but you can also live well with it."
>
> —songbird

> "It's such a strange thing to have 'how are you' be such a loaded question."
>
> —webfoot45

A friend of mine, who was going through some awful times at the same time as me, told me what you should say when people ask "how are you" in that drippy way. She told me to say "fine" with a big smile. You know what f-i-n-e stands for? *F***ed up, insecure, neurotic,* and *exhausted.* Not the nicest sentiment, but saying that has helped me to smile at some very difficult people.

    webfoot45

Worst comment: from my husband who, when they removed the bandages, said, "Oh, look, Bride of Frankenstein." I'll never forget that moment.

    Extreme Self Care

Sometimes I would rather hear "how are you" than nothing. There are so many people who just don't ask me how I am doing. I do not know if it is fear of my response or not knowing what to say. I appreciate the "how are you" because at least they are trying to keep up with me.

    Kellyk01

I had a very "dear" friend that told me that if I had to get cancer that at least I was "lucky" and got breast cancer. I asked her why she thought I was lucky and she replied, "Well, isn't it the most easy to treat?" Now I wouldn't call chemo, throwing up, having massive pain, not being able to catch my breath, 6 surgeries in 3 months, severe exhaustion, and sometimes not being able to even get out of bed for lack of energy being "lucky." What was this girl thinking??

    Irish Nana

One of my favorite lines has been, "So, are you all recovered now?" As if! (Though that line isn't nearly as good as, "What's your prognosis?")

I try to appreciate that most of the questions and comments are well-meaning, but honestly folks, it makes me wonder sometimes.

oceanwalker

I struggle with the "how are you?" questions all the time because many people don't realize I have metastatic cancer and will never be done with treatment. Very few people have ever heard of someone surviving late-stage breast cancer, let alone have thought of it as a potentially "chronic" as opposed to acute disease. So I often wonder whether to tell them when they ask how I am feeling; do they even know I am still full of cancer, even if it is stable? Even friends who have had Stage I or II cancers sometimes seem surprised that I am still on active treatment. Mostly I just say I am fine so far and leave it at that; it can be too hard to explain.

Every time I get my hair cut now my hairdresser says a prayer under her breath for me and for herself. I think by living our normal lives and being out in the community we are examples to people that you can get cancer, but you can also live well with it. I rely on my best friends and my husband when I am feeling down from someone's comments, but usually I shrug them off—I can control my reaction even if I can't control their questions, and almost all of them mean well.

songbird

People assume that every mistake I make and that every time I am tired or out of sorts has to do with breast cancer. Even three years later, when I say I don't feel well, almost everyone I know gets that really concerned look on their faces, and that "oh dear" tone in their voices. I'm fine! I just have a headache!

webfoot45

I find it a double-edged sword as to people asking how I am. I appreciate their concern, however when they screw up their face and say, "Are you sure, are you really sure?" then it gets me upset as it seems like I have to stop and ask my chemo-fogged brain: I am okay, right??

> lucky7

Years ago going through breast cancer treatments, I had lost some weight; a friend saw me in the local diner and remarked, "Hey, you've lost some weight, you look good." Rather than thank him, what came right out of my mouth was "Yes, breast cancer can do that to you." He was speechless. Don't know what came over me!

> betty

I had a physical therapist helping me learn lymphedema massage and we were talking about the Team in Training events she had run where she raised money for cancer research. And then she said that she had to take a break because she got all "cancered out." Hmm. Wish I could take a break from being all cancered out.

> LukesMom

From a favorite aunt: "Don't worry, only the good die young." Really. And I'm sitting there thinking, "Wait! I'm GOOD! What does that mean???" People don't know what to say and instead of being quiet they feel the need to say something. "Something" is often *stupid*. But that comment was 16 years ago and I never stopped loving her.

> deb

CHAPTER NINE

Mothers and Daughters

"When I told my mom about my diagnosis, she cried and apologized as if it was something she gave me."

Dee

Once a woman has cancer, the bond between mother and daughter is immediately impacted. Rarely did the women feel things remained the same with their mothers—regardless of their age—and not one woman was bland or indifferent in her assessment. Some women report that their relationships are greatly reinforced, others that they are sadly strained. Often, the role of the caretaker shifts, with the adult daughter now protecting her aging mother. But the traditional role of mother-as-protector is just as deeply desired, as expressed by the woman who writes that her mother "was the only woman that [I] wanted to share this scary worry with." Compare this with the unsympathetic mother who said her daughter's cancer was "just a blip on the radar screen." Given how much I had on my mind and the decisions I was considering just after diagnosis, I was grateful that my mother managed to keep her cool around me. It was exactly what I needed. But if you were to ask my closest friends *how she felt, you'd get a different picture: worried, watchful, and wary. No wonder: not only am I the youngest of three children, I'm also the only girl, which raised the emotional ante between my mother and me. Like many women here, my cancer brought us closer.*

An especially heartfelt group was those women whose mothers once had breast cancer; none of them were angry at their mothers but instead they experienced deep empathy with what their mothers had long ago experienced. And another kind of heartache: the woman who wanted to protect her aged mother, a Holocaust survivor, from learning that she had cancer. Many women spoke of their own young daughters, wondering how to safeguard their future against breast cancer. For the woman who has two primary relationships—as daughter and as parent—the dynamic is especially poignant.

GENERATION OF GIRLS

I am wondering how many of you with living mothers and/or daughters have found that breast cancer is a catalyst for increasing your connection and maybe overcoming some of the natural communication barriers that seem to exist once we all grow up. I have always been close to my 76-year-old mom and this has brought us even closer; we are telling each other things about ourselves, our dreams, and feelings that we might have ignored before. I am blessed to have such a wonderful mom, and I know this has been very hard for her.
    songbird

I was having an extremely difficult time with my mother when I was diagnosed with breast cancer seven years ago. My mother had recently gone through a difficult transition with both her physical and mental health. She was in her late 60s at the time and I was mid-40s. Both of our hard times brought us closer together. The little things don't bother us at all. I heard my mother remark the other day that she is happier now than she has been her entire life! She has remarked that now that she's learned how to live, she can think easier about the dying. She has normal aging aches and pains of a 70ish female, but she's much happier. As am I.

The relationship with my daughter who was 9 when I was diagnosed and is now 16 (!) has incurred some of the natural turmoil of a mom with an adolescent daughter. After my mastectomy and reconstruction, it took me at least 2 years to get undressed fully in front of her. Now we share dressing rooms together and laugh at our "goofy" ever-changing figures. (Hers for the better! Mine is going way south!) She doesn't comment, snicker, or feel sorry for her mom. Her mom (just) survived cancer and that's why she looks different. My daughter will tell people that I'm basically the same, probably better . . . and I would agree.

Stormy

My mother and I have a sometimes strained relationship and she has at times been very critical of me, other times hovering and worrying to the point I withheld telling her things. Currently she is 82 years old and somewhat forgetful; I have not expected much motherly nurturing from her for years. When I told her of my diagnosis, she was quite distressed, and since we live several hours from each other, it was hard. She was more upset than I expected, and still, 8 months later, asks, "How *are* you?" and when I answer "Fine," she says, *"Really?"* She has lots of cosmetic concerns anyway, so it's hard to talk about things like body image and changes, etc., with her. I just don't.

My mother-in-law has been my mom by function since I married her son 17 years ago. She is just great, so it was extremely hard to tell her about my diagnosis too. She is a very strong Christian, and her faith has helped to strengthen mine. Mom is 84 now, and someone with whom I can discuss anything, including my fears about my own mortality. I know she talks to me about very personal things too, and I feel honored.

I also have a daughter who is 33 tomorrow, lovely inside and out, with a daughter of her own. My granddaughter was 6 months old when I was diagnosed, and it is incredibly painful for me to think of these generations of mine possibly someday being affected by breast cancer. My daughter and I have talked a lot about my breast cancer. For a while we were afraid of my dying, but now we focus more on the present and cherish each other in this moment in time.

Lizzi

When I told my mom about my diagnosis, she cried and apologized as if it was something she gave me. There was no breast cancer in my family history before my diagnosis. I was very close with my mom and 2 younger sisters. I am the oldest of 5. My mother had double bypass heart surgery 7 years before me. She lived 15 years after her surgery. She died August 2002 and I miss her love and support, even though the last couple of years Alzheimer's was getting the best of her.

As for my 2 daughters, who were 14 and 19 when I went through all this, they too were strong young girls and I know I leaned on them for help. I am blessed with these women who take on disease like soldiers going into battle.

Dee

All of my family is long distance. I'm in South Carolina, my mom is in Texas. She has been very supportive, in her own way. My mom had breast cancer 10 years ago, but caught it so early she just had to have surgery, no chemo or radiation. The fact that she and my sister are RNs is a plus. I haven't seen her since all this started, but she's going to try to come out for a week after I have recuperated somewhat from my reconstruction. We've never been especially close; she's not one of those huggy-kissy mothers, and I don't think she's ever said "I love you," but that's just the way she is.

kathi1964

YOU AND YOUR DAUGHTER

My daughter and I have always been close. She is my best friend and I am her best friend. My getting this disease has been extremely hard on her. We lost her dad to stomach cancer 16 years ago when she was only 10. I know that my daughter thinks about it all the time.

NMRose

My daughter is 18 and just graduated from high school. She was 14 when I was diagnosed. During my surgeries and chemo she was somewhat distant and seemed slightly angry with me. It hurt me at the time, but I love her so much. Each year she walks with me in the Relay for Life. This year the relay was on the same evening as her prom and I didn't think she would make it. But she walked with me in her prom dress and got a lot of praise from bystanders. I was so proud of her.

I want her to take her breast health seriously and to some extent she does take the whole breast cancer awareness thing very seriously, but she's young and you know how young people thing they're invincible.

sapphire

"According to my daughter, it is a mother's primary goal in life to drive her children insane. Apparently I'm quite good at it :)"

kathi1964

I am the mom with breast cancer and I found out some interesting thoughts from my daughter. I live in a small town and know darn near everyone; with that being said, many are acquaintances but not close friends. My daughter works in a restaurant in town and is 22. We had a good chat the other day about how this is affecting her. My daughter started to cry as she told me how difficult this has been for her, especially through her shifts at work.

She said to me, "Mom do you know what it is like to have to tell people up to 10 times a day how your mother is?" She said, "I am at home, and you are there. I think about the breast cancer, I go to work, and people are constantly asking me about you. I can't get away from it, not even at work!!!"

I hugged her and we both cried for a bit and then I said, "How about if I come to work with you and sit in the middle of the room on a chair? Then when people ask you, you can say there she is!! Viewing and questions will be between 2 P.M. and 4 P.M." We had a chuckle about it all.

My daughter had also commented to me at the beginning, "I don't want a broken Mom. Moms are supposed to fix us, not the other way around." I know she didn't mean I was *broken* broken, but rather it was a statement of hers and the families feeling of helplessness in this whole situation.

Moms are supposed to make everyone feel alright; when we get breast cancer or any illness the ripple effects through the family are endless.

Dragonfli

> "I want her to take her breast health seriously and to some extent she does take the whole breast cancer awareness thing very seriously, but she's young and you know how young people think they're invincible."
>
> sapphire

GROWING CLOSER TO YOUR MOTHER

When I finally told my mother about my upcoming biopsy, she insisted on coming with me. She took me home afterward, got me into bed, and then burst into tears. Apparently she felt that it was her "fault" that I'd gotten breast cancer because she and her mother had both had breast cancer 20+ years earlier. I reassured her that nothing was her fault and that I had no such feelings about it. Heredity is heredity, not something one can foist upon another.

abrenner

> "My mom has turned into my closest friend."
>
> webfoot45

My mother is a very active, healthy woman. She was 68 at the time of my diagnosis and I was 39. Our relationship has been loving but strained at times. We are both independent and somewhat controlling women, which doesn't always make for a harmonious relationship. I am also a very private person and she's a bit of a busybody. I know that it took a great deal of effort for my mother to respect my privacy and need to be independent during surgery, treatment, and since, but she did. I know she wanted to come with me to all of my treatments but I just didn't want it to be a big drama. My compromise was to ask her to come to my first treatment so she could see I was fine and then I did the rest on my own.

I have a new respect for my mom as a human being after this experience because she was able to really behave as a person who truly loves another. She was able to put my needs before her own even if that meant not being as involved in this difficult time as she would have liked to have been. We are closer today for the experience.

uneven but breathin

> "I knew my mom would be there if I needed her and she learned I'd ask for help when I needed it."
>
> uneven but breathin

My mother and I have never really been close. She tended to favor my brothers more than her girls for some reason. When I was diagnosed, this changed. My mother told me, for the very first time in 37 years, that she loved me going into the surgery room. I was *totally shocked*! This is a word that she doesn't use at all. I love the relationship that we share now—2 years and going strong.

flyingwithoutwings

> "I realized that as much as I had to let my mother in for my own needs, I also was given the gift of helping her to heal in some ways."
>
> abrenner

My mom seemed to be the only person in my life that could put their own feelings aside enough to let me vent mine. What I didn't anticipate was that after my treatment, when she went back to her house and to her life, that I couldn't turn that intimacy off. It took me some time to get used to, that our relationship could never go back to the comfortable distance I was used to, but now it is a huge blessing. My mom has turned into my closest friend.

webfoot45

> "My mother was the only woman that I wanted to share this scary worry with because we were so close."
>
> Eileen

MOTHERS ARE MIXED BAGS

My mother has good intentions, or at least I like to believe that. Regardless, I love her; I just don't always like her.

kimmytoo

This is a complicated one. There's so much to say but the point I want to highlight is that my mom wasn't very supportive during treatment. The support I received from my mom was very skin deep, maybe in part because she just didn't know what to do. My mom came for 2 of the surgeries for a day or two. When she came she was helpful.

When treatment was over, my mom had the attitude of "well, glad that's over with." She didn't understand how I had changed, and didn't want to. The pitiful thing is that shortly after my treatment ended, my dad was diagnosed with colon cancer. My mom immediately treated his cancer as much more life-threatening which bothered me because I was Stage III/IV—I guess she just didn't get it. Unfortunately she was right, because after 5 months of suffering through dreadful unsuccessful treatments, my dad died. My dad and I weren't particularly close so missing him doesn't bring my mom and I closer but we are closer now because I think she finally gets it. I'm sure sorry she had to learn this way.

Anne M.

> "I get the sense that difficult mothers were always difficult and that breast cancer just brings it into focus in a more maddening way."
>
> MCN

My mother has never been emotionally demonstrative, and although I've learned to accept that she's not going to be physically affectionate or say "I love you," I'm very disappointed that she can't reach out to me and be supportive at the most difficult time in my life. When I was first diagnosed, I tried to talk to her on the phone about being scared of surgery, chemo, etc. After listening for a couple of minutes, she said "Okay, now let's talk about something upbeat." I didn't expect her to be a shoulder to cry on, but she doesn't even know what my treatment schedule is, even though I've told her repeatedly. I'm not angry, just very sad.

Towanda2

> "Do they really set out to drive us as crazy as they do, or can our mothers just annoy us quicker than anyone on earth?"
>
> dreambeliever

> "I've learned that family of choice is just as powerful as family of origin."
>
> solucky

My mother has always been a very sick and unhealthy person; she complains constantly, but never stops going and doing things for others for fear she will really be down if she ever quits (we tend to never give up, one of the few things we have in common). My breast cancer has always been devastating for her and now that I have metastatic breast cancer, she has just zoned out concerning the facts and believes every treatment I receive "cures" me a little more. She still worries constantly about me, but just doesn't get it that this time around it may be chronic for a while, but not curable. I just let her believe whatever, if that is the way she has to cope, I understand.

dreambeliever

"MOMMY DEAREST"

Boy, is this a touchy subject. My mother is a true narcissist, so my cancer was either something to bring attention to her or something to compete with for attention. I know that sounds harsh, but that's how it is. While it is sad (and I am grateful to the cancer experience for allowing me to see this at 30 instead of 50 or 60), I have compassion for her. However, we are for the most part estranged. When I told her about my recurrence she said, "It's just a blip on the radar screen." I believe that if cancer doesn't serve as a wake-up call, it usually just brings out more of the same in a person, for better or worse. On the other hand, I have met some wonderful mother-figures who have been extremely kind and supportive. I've learned that family of choice is just as powerful as family of origin.

solucky

My mom and I had a close relationship for years. About the time I was diagnosed, she began dating. She'd been widowed for 15 years, and swore she'd never date, but she was like a giddy teenager when she finally made the leap. Anyway, while I was in the hospital for a week after my surgery, my mom only came to see me twice! The hospital was 15 minutes from her house, and she was retired and active. The second time, she asked if she could bring her new beau whom I hadn't met yet, and I said no, I wasn't in any condition to meet someone new. I think at that point she made the choice to go with the beau instead of me, and basically began avoiding me.

Now my mom has advanced stage Alzheimer's disease and I'm the decision maker, authority in her life. Good thing I don't hold a grudge, huh!?

Janet

I have *never* been sick in my life, always very healthy and vibrant. On the other hand, my mother has had emphysema for about a decade (she is 71, I am 36). For quite some time now, she had been the only "sick one" and she is not a very upbeat sick, either, but a very pessimistic "woe is me" kind of sick person.

I noticed the "problem" first when I had my surgery. My parents and my sister (she is a nurse, and she stayed with me for a week to help with the drains) were with me, both at the hospital and at home. I was inundated with visitors, gifts, flowers, phone calls, etc. I have a fabulous bunch of friends and colleagues. Well, I started to notice that my mother appeared jealous of all the attention I was getting. She kept trying to turn the conversation or the attention to herself and her illness. Needless to say, I was flabbergasted.

As the weeks passed, and I went through chemo, I would talk to her about different things, like trying to eat, etc. Always, she would turn the conversation around so it was about her emphysema, and how difficult it was for her, blah blah blah. She made it like it was a contest about who could be the sickest! Well, guess what, she can have the title! Sometimes I feel like screaming at her that I didn't choose to get breast cancer, that I didn't do anything to get it, that my case is tragic, as opposed to her emphysema, which is a direct result of the fact that she smoked for 5 decades! This is a sensitive subject for me. Now I feel like I have a fractured relationship with my mother. I used to speak with her every day, and for some reason, when I wasn't sick, her constant moaning didn't get to me and I would commiserate. Now, I just can't take her.

SusieQ

SusieQ, my mom and I are the same ages as you and your mom. Dealing with the cancer thing with my mom has been interesting, as she was a few years' survivor of Stage III lung cancer at the time of my diagnosis. I found that I just couldn't tell my mother I had cancer, so I got my sister to do it. She would find a way to make this about her, yet this was about me.

She was less demanding during the time I had cancer, yet as soon as I was done with treatment she was on my case about visiting more often, etc. Heck, one time when I was going through chemo, she was so busy telling me about her own health concerns that she forgot to ask how I was.

Our relationship was never good, but after using my own cancer experience to help others and seeing her milk her experience for her own benefit whenever possible just makes me lose all respect.

bradleyteach

My mother, the drama queen

My thing is that my mom has used me for attention from coworkers, etc. I *hate* it! I live 6 hours away and still catch wind of some of her stories. I had a big scare about 2 months ago with some bone scans and such showing some spots. My brother calls me and tells me that my mom has called my dad (and grandma!) and said that they found spots in my lungs and that I'm going to die. I don't get it.

I love her, and I know that she will always be right here when I need her, but the *drama* that comes with it makes it so hard. I have to screen the info that I give her or I risk it going awry to others, it's so silly. It's like I'm the adult in the relationship.

kimmytoo

WHEN YOUR MOTHER IS NO LONGER LIVING

I wish my mother was alive. She passed away eight months before I was diagnosed with breast cancer. She had fought the disease herself. Her mother fought the disease as well. I wanted to be hugged by her and comforted by her. My mother was a wise and sensitive lady who was respected and admired by many. She had taught me about illness and how to be knowledgeable so whatever it is can be addressed in the most effective and practical manner. Unfortunately, there was a lot of illness in my family, ranging from my father to my sister to my grandmother to my mother, so hospitals and doctors were not feared, but rather seen as hope, a positive force. I was not afraid when I was diagnosed thanks to my mother.

Jacquie

When I was diagnosed I remember being glad, in this single instance, that my mother was no longer alive. My mom and I were very close and it would have been extraordinarily difficult to tell her about my breast cancer. I'm happy she was spared that knowledge and the fear it would have brought her.

pennywise

My mom died one week after I found the lump in my breast while showering at her home as I took care of her in her final days (she died of a primary lung cancer that followed her breast cancer diagnosis 23 years prior). I knew that I could not share my fear that the breast mass I felt probably was cancerous due to our family history with this disease. This was difficult and easy at the same time. I needed to protect her from any additional worry and make her last days free from distraction so that she could focus on how we could meet her needs. That was the easy part. The hard part was that she was the only woman that I wanted to share this scary worry with. I missed my mother at that time and I wondered what she experienced when she felt her own breast mass in 1961, when *no one* talked about breast cancer.

Eileen

Playwright's mother was a Holocaust survivor

At first my mother was in complete denial. Even in the hospital, she refused to believe I was there for my tumor to be removed. She was a Holocaust survivor, an observant Jew, who always believed that somehow God was looking after her. She couldn't reconcile her view of the world with God giving me cancer. Her friends told me that she prayed for me every day. We hardly ever spoke about it, but she was as helpful as she could be, helping me with my own two young daughters at the time (1 and 3), although she was 80.

I always admired my mother because I never thought I could have survived what she went through in Europe. I always thought I would simply shrivel up and die of fear if anything like that were fac-ing me. But whatever she was made of, I got a fair dose of it, and it held me in good stead when I was going through treatment. I always spoke up for myself, asked every question, and often thought of her as I moved through these difficult years. I have always been uncomfort-able with the word "survivor" because for me, as a first-generation Jew in America, my parents were the true survivors.

My mother passed away almost five years ago. When she died her friends told me that she used to sit on her porch every day and read prayers just for me. When I drive by her old house, I can still see her rocking in that old chair of hers.

playwright

CHAPTER TEN

Children

"I am a very proud mother and leaving this
world right now is just not an option."

Jackjoy

As many times as I have read these stories, the tears come easily. I shake my head, I sigh over the pathos expressed here, I applaud the courage. This most primal of bonds—mother and child—is also the most wrenching of relationships for a woman who has breast cancer. Consider these questions raised by the women: Would they be around to see their children grow up? If not, who would mother their children? And how the hell do you prepare yourself to die, knowing your children will suffer? How will you be remembered? How do you protect your child when you are sick, much less get a meal on the table or go over homework together? How do you handle the guilt of not "being there" as a parent, of missing a basketball game or birthday party? For women with daughters, there is the nagging question, have their daughters inherited this disease? And how do you respond to your child's tears or, worse, what should you do when your child shuts down and turns away from you? Just how resilient are children?

Mercifully, there are silver linings in these dark clouds. Adversity brings out togetherness, and adversity also teaches compassion. The *mother with young children, the mother with grown children, the woman who still someday hopes to be a mother, the woman who will never be able to have a child because of her disease . . . these are cries from the battlefield that echo in the home of every woman dealing with breast cancer.*

> "The gift of time is the best Mother's Day gift ever."
>
> lambda77

ALL IN THE FAMILY

Some of us get our diagnosis when our children are very young. I did—mine were 4 and 12. There is nothing more difficult than choosing between doing something to save your life, and being totally present for your children and their normal needs. In a zillion ways this has been my dilemma for 15 years. My kids remember that I stopped making homemade ice cream when I got cancer. And there are multitudes of such instances.

That's the rub. There's no way to be the best mother we can be, the mother we want to be, and also do the best and most right thing for getting rid of our breast cancer and regaining our health. It is a deeply wrenching conflict. Mothers with cancer have the toughest row to hoe.

Susana

> "You aren't the only one on that rollercoaster ride when you have breast cancer. Your family members ride with you whether they want to or not."
>
> Dee

I wanted life to be as normal as possible for my children, so my parents and my husband went to every school event, play, classroom presentation. That was great for the kids and helped me a lot. I've been "sick" all of their lives, and often very, very sick. I'm a pretty optimistic person and I hope that attitude has helped them. What I've seen with my kids is that they always wanted Mommy to be fine and then it was "let's move on to *me*." And that's the way it should be. One last thing: I always knew they loved me, but I also knew they had to be children first. So I let go, let my parents fill in, and let my kids grow and learn. I think it's been an important lesson for all of us. Made me a better parent.

deb

> "My kids remember that I stopped making homemade ice cream when I got cancer. And there are multitudes of such instances."
>
> Susana

I have two beautiful sons that have spent their entire life with a mother who has advanced breast cancer. I used to think this was such a negative thing as I felt like I had spoiled their childhood. I now look at them 9 years and 10 years old and see that they have become the most special little people with an insight far beyond their years.

They know that I may not be around when they grow up so they give me more cuddles (they suggested my "code" name here) than most of their peers give their mothers. My eldest son sometimes looks me in the eyes at bedtime and it is as if he is making a mental picture of me to hold on to forever. I have two reasons that I keep going to have treatment every week and they are my children. I love them more than anything on this earth and I will do whatever it takes to keep me on this earth.

Cuddles

My 2 teenage daughters are the main reason that I have agreed to go through so much to live. There have been many times that I just wanted to quit my treatments and they were so supportive and there for me in every way that I just closed my eyes and dragged my feet and kept moving forward. We have such a special and close relationship that has been enhanced because of my cancer.

newday

TELLING YOUR CHILDREN: "I HAVE CANCER . . ."

I have a son who is turning 6 this month, and two girls who are 8 and 9. This was sooo hard on them at first, because they thought that I was going to die right then, as soon as we told them that I had cancer. (My uncle just died from lung cancer a year before, and I didn't realize that they would make the connection.) After a couple of months, I finally figured out that I needed to tell them that even though I may die from this someday, I would be able to let them know because my doctors would be able to tell me. That helped them tremendously, knowing that I would keep them in the loop. We don't keep secrets, because their imagination is way worse than the truth.

kimmytoo

> "Keep communication open and hope for the best."
>
> artistic person

I remember the day that I told my children. My daughter was 6 and my son 3. It was one of the hardest days of my life. My daughter had some emotional breakdowns throughout my treatment because I wasn't able to spend the time with her that she so loved. My husband was extremely supportive but stressed himself trying to run his business, take care of the kids and me. My son on the other hand is my baby. He had a really hard time. It was his first year in preschool and he knew in his heart that I was really sick. He cried every day for the first five months of school. As I was getting further and further into treatment he started getting used to it and now I see happiness in his eyes again. I see my daughter laughing and I just want to cry. I feel that even though I had no control over getting cancer I have put such a burden on my husband and my kids to deal with. I am the one who should be taking care of them, not the other way around. It is just so frustrating. I want my life back and I don't think it will ever be back the way I want it.

littleone

I just told my nearly 9-year-old daughter after obsessing for 5 years about when and how to tell her. Her big concern: can you catch it from someone who has it.

Annie

My 12-year-old immediately started crying when I said I had cancer because "cancer kills." I realized that we tell kids at a very young age that smoking causes cancer, and cancer kills. So most kids associate cancer with death automatically.

kathi1964

When my husband and I received my breast cancer confirmation from my doctor, the thing that finally made me break down was asking the doctor, "How do I tell my children?" He didn't have an answer for me and all I could do was cry. We waited until the weekend to tell them and in the meantime I spoke with other people who had to explain medical or traumatic events to their children and got some good advice. My boys are 7 and 9. We were advised not to make a big event of the news as that makes it scarier and never comes off as planned.

We simply explained my upcoming surgery and the medicine that I would get, how my hair would fall out and I'd be sick some of the time. We explained that they would need to help out some more and so would Dad. Then we just answered their questions. My nine-year-old immediately asked if I was going to die—out of the mouths of babes. That was hard. We told him no. My prognosis was very good; it was early so it wasn't a stretch. In hindsight, I think we may have downplayed it a little too much. I was hoping for a little more empathy from them, but I can keep working on that.

They kept asking questions randomly, at the bus stop, over dinner, etc. We always answered as truthfully as possible. We also told their teachers at school and the parents of some of their closest friends, knowing that kids talk and they'd probably see me bald.

Michele

NURTURING INDEPENDENCE

My children were 4 and 6 when I was diagnosed. I was upfront with them by saying that I had cancer and explained that there would be surgery and medicine that would make my hair fall out. They needed reassurance that I wasn't going to die from this as my mom had died from cancer 2 years earlier.

What helped my family was that I was the first of my sisters to be diagnosed. I did very well, so when they were diagnosed their children could see that while things would be different, the outcome could be okay.

What changed the most was that I wanted to be sure my kids would do well without me, if need be, and helped them towards independence at a very early age. I was always there and we are close, but after watching my sisters and me in chemo, they had to learn to do a lot for themselves. I think sometimes that I may have pushed them too far away too soon, but I needed to know that they would be able to take care of themselves.

lambda77

This has been a big struggle. I tried to minimize things and hide my fear from my children. And I also have seen my job as their comforter, and have not allowed them to assume the role of my comforter. My kids are 9, 12, and 15. I don't know if this is right or wrong. But I do know that they have pretty much carried on their lives as if the only thing different was I had no hair. They place the same expectations on me to make dinner, do the laundry, listen to their complaints, break up their arguments. On one hand I am thankful that my family doesn't cater to my cancer. But on the other hand, I wonder if my façade of strength hasn't disabled them from having sympathy for me?

 highaim

Isn't it amazing how resilient children are? We made a "Happy Helper" chore list and I was surprised and delighted at the skills my family learned to do. It might not have been the way I did these things or as good as I could do them but they were proud to help and this made them feel like they were taking some control over the situation.

 Eve

The first time I was diagnosed, my kids (from a previous marriage) were 12 and 10. We pretty much told them everything, and they went and met with the doctors a couple of times with us. I felt they needed to be prepared for the effects of chemo, radiation, etc. Of course it wasn't easy, but they seemed to deal with it okay. My son, who was 10 at the time, would come in the bathroom while I was puking my guts out during chemo and massage my head, or put a cold wash cloth on the back of my neck. By the time I was diagnosed the second time, I had a 16-month-old who, of course, didn't understand much. By the third time, my daughter was 5 and I then had a 5-month-old. We tried explaining to her in simple terms what cancer was, why they had removed my breasts, and what would happen during chemo. One day she commented that, "Well, I guess when I become a mom I'll have to have the same thing done." Needless to say, that broke my heart.

 I felt it was important that my children know everything and realize that I may need them and their help sometimes. That's was families are for—to help each other. Sometimes I think it made them feel a little less helpless. They couldn't take away the cancer, but they could help me get through it.

little jumper

BRAVERY COMES IN SMALL SIZES, TOO

At the local (breast cancer) races each year my children love to go and race in the tot trot. This year my son moved up a level to the kids for the cure. He was the youngest in his new age group. He raced really hard. Later he said to me, "Mommy, I wanted to win the race for you because whoever wins the race does their mommy never get breast cancer again?" I know children follow your cues, but their strength and child wisdom have been gifts to me.

jonessugar

> "Without knowing it, cancer gave my daughter character."
>
> smilie

My daughter is 11 now; she was 8 when I was diagnosed. She was actually with me (so was my mother) when I got the word that I had cancer. My initial reaction was just to weep like a baby for what seemed like a very long time. She was right there beside me, rubbing my back, telling me not to cry; even now it's hard to think about. I sometimes wish that I had been able to be stronger since she was there in the room, but how do you control a reaction from your heart like that?

Last year she had to write an essay about who she admired most and why, and she wrote it about me and my battle with breast cancer. I kept it of course and every time I read it, I cry all over again. I know this hasn't been easy on anyone in my family, but for my daughter it's probably been the hardest and I am so proud of her for the way she has handled herself through it all.

Maryegkh

The proudest moment was when my daughter showed me her college application essay: "My life has changed—for the better—since my mother had breast cancer." She went on to say how seeing me suffer and survive made her a better person. She has seen how family working together creates a special bond. Her outlook on life is to take the challenges and make them her own. Without knowing it, cancer gave my daughter character.

smilie

My children were 1 and 3 when I was diagnosed. When the doctor gave me the news that I had cancer I was with my mom and sister. My mom had breast cancer 22 years earlier at the age of 31. I remember being terribly afraid for my mom when she was so sick. I was old enough to remember how bad things were for her. Anyway, on way the home from the doctor's office I begged my mom and sister not to let my kids see me sick. I wanted them to be sheltered from this horrific disease. When I got home I took my 3-year-old to the side and with tears in my eyes I told her that I had some bad news. I asked her to please help me by helping to take care of her baby sister. When I returned home from the hospital after having a bilateral mastectomy my two little girls came up to me and asked me if I was okay and that they missed me. Then they started to kiss my hands and rub my arms (I used to do that to them when they were sick). My oldest girl told me that she took very good care of her sister and asked me if I was proud of her. My heart soared. That was the best medicine I could have ever gotten. I may not have approached the subject in the best way with my babies but I did the best that I could.

KerryMcD

My daughter was 5 when I was diagnosed and went through my surgery. (She is now almost 14.) I don't remember exactly when I told my daughter about my diagnosis but I do remember when I came home with drains from my surgery that she got into the shower with me one day to hold them because she thought they were going to fall out. This little girl not only had a mom who had breast cancer, she had a dad who only a month before had triple bypass surgery.

Joanne

What do you say to the two most important people in your life? I fought for these kids—3 life-threatening pregnancies, my son nearly died when both lungs collapsed at birth, my daughter fought a horrible illness at birth and I lost a baby between. We have been a family of survivors. Cancer took away their innocence and taught them more about fear than they had ever experienced.

My son is 16 now and life has pretty much gone back to normal for him. To me it seemed like my cancer was in the past for him until the last few weeks. His last report in class was on breast cancer. This 16-year-old boy stood up in front of his peers and put together a power point presentation on breast cancer. I was so deeply touched. He got an A by the way.

Princess86

My children were 14, 13, and 8 at the time of my diagnosis. And believe me, their reactions were as different from each other as could be. My husband and I sat our oldest two down first and told them everything and were very straightforward about it all. My daughter (14) reacted first with terror and then within a few minutes, she got up and ran over to her best friend's house. From then on, she was very flippant about my situation. My feelings were very hurt, but I let her "do her thing." The interesting part was that about 2 months later, I found out that her English teacher had entered a composition she had written into a literary fair in our area and it eventually wound up taking first place in the state of Missouri for all 9th (she was) and 10th graders. Wow!! It was the most profound and heart-wrenching thing I have ever read. It included everything she had been going through from my diagnosis ("what if mom dies") to my surgery ("I now have to become the mother and take care of the family while mom can't"), to dealing with her family ("I can't bear to look into my father's eyes and see the pain as he tries to be strong for all of us"). I had no idea she had had so many feelings pent-up inside and how eloquently she could express them.

maumau66

SO MANY QUESTIONS, SO FEW PERFECT ANSWERS

I have been blessed with two healthy little (not so little anymore) girls. One is 8 and the other 13. I will admit that my very biggest fear about being diagnosed was leaving my children without a mother. My father died in his sleep suddenly when he was 51 (I was 25) and I fear that more than anything. My oldest would ask me several times if I was going to die. I didn't want to tell her no since I could not know this and yet you have to be so creative about your answers. I never wanted to die and have her tell others that I lied to her.

Krista

> "Children are the most honest and accepting humans."
>
> sibling rivalry

My 8-year-old daughter was told separately from the big kids and in a way an 8-year-old could understand things. Her biggest fear was my surgery. She worried a lot about me when I was not myself: after surgery, the week after chemo, and especially when I lost my hair. She wants to understand everything and keeps asking if "the cancer is

gone." I tell her yes, because that's the simple answer, although I
know it's much more complicated than that. She has trouble going to
sleep some nights and wants me to lay with her at which time she asks
me the same questions over and over: "Is the cancer gone?", "Will it
come back ever?", "Can kids get cancer?", and the most painful
one—"Did she do something wrong to make me get cancer?" Of
course I very strongly told her that it was not possible for that to happen and that we don't know why I got cancer, at which time she asks
again if we don't know why, then could it come back and could she get
it. It's the same thing over and over again every night. It's hard to be
a psychologist with your own children. It's so personal.

maumau66

One day I got in the tub with my son (he was only 16 months old
when I was diagnosed). He looked at my chest and pointed to my
breast and said "Boobie." Then he looked at my mastectomy scar and
said "Mommy, where Boobie?" I looked at him and told him "It is in
the drawer." His response? "Okay, play toys now!" I guess they are
resilient too.

Max's Mommy

WHO'S THE ROLE MODEL: YOU OR YOUR CHILDREN?

We have a 15-year-old son, and 12-year-old daughter. Last summer
when I told our son I have to have a mastectomy, he replied "that
sucks." Initially I was hurt that he didn't respond with something else
and he didn't care, but I later realized he had no idea what exactly a
"mastectomy" meant, what it looked like, how it would effect his mother
emotionally, etc. He certainly has learned a lot, and has seen me sobbing at the loss of my right breast last summer and my left 4 weeks ago.
And guess what—he was there to hug and comfort me, and reassure
me "that breasts don't make a woman, Mom!", caring for me when I
was recovering, bringing me food and drinks in bed and snuggling up

and watching TV with me in bed so I wasn't alone. For a young man, he too has probably learned far more than he even realizes, until the time comes that he has a serious relationship with a woman.

Big Red

> "I have two reasons that I keep going to have treatment every week and they are my children."
>
> Cuddles

My daughter is almost 4 and she knows I am battling the "Cancer Monster." She is so young to have to worry that Mama isn't feeling well; she tells me when I need to rest. I do not want her youthfulness/purity to be overwhelmed by cancer. I nursed her for $2\frac{1}{2}$ years; my breasts were/are the thing she wants to be next to when she is scared or hurt. The other day when I was posting about the angst of my scarred breast she crawled into my lap and out of the blue said "I like your boobies, Mama." She may spend couch time for this love, but she makes me see beyond the angst my breasts and the cancer they hosted brought me and helps curtail my vanity about them.

Mamaper

CHILDREN AND SCHOOL

I remember when my son, who was in 2nd grade at the time, came home from school in a funk. When I asked what was wrong he denied anything. After a little probing and calling some friends, I learned that the reading specialist in his school had died due to complications from lung cancer. The school took it upon themselves to hold a memorial service during the school day for everyone. The students had no choice in whether they wanted to attend. Since there was no notice sent home about this (can you imagine?), my son had to sit through a service at the age of 8 listening to all the wonderful things this teacher had done. Afterward, when I got him to talk about it (I mean *cry* about it), he told me how frightened he was because this woman had cancer and I also had cancer. He put 2 and 2 together and figured that I was going to die. Lesson here: we can never prepare our children's schools enough about our diagnosis and the impact that might occur when others around receive a similar diagnosis.

Eileen

THE UPS AND DOWNS OF PREGNANCY AND WANTING MORE CHILDREN

> "I never realized what a big part cancer had in stopping a woman from having children until I got breast cancer."
>
> pinkwings

I found out I was pregnant with my 3rd child 6 months after I finished my cancer treatments. My doctors were *very* positive about it. I am 34 and did not think I wanted more kids until the test came back positive. But now I am thrilled and my other kids are thrilled. I never had a chance to have a follow-up mammogram after treatment (got pregnant before it could happen) so it will be 15 months from end of treatment before I can get one again. That makes me a little nervous. But I feel like this was meant to be.

Francesca

"I really wanted to have a baby (I'm not at all interested in a career) and it's amazingly difficult to have all that washed away. Frankly,

I'm more sad about that than I was about the cancer. . . . it was easier to deal with the idea of not having a life than it is to deal with the
idea of having a life without purpose."

alleeum

Infertility

These three women discuss the real pain of not being fertile because of their disease.

> "I was expected to just be thankful that my
> cancer was stabilized for the time being, but
> how can I fully appreciate that when at the
> same time all my dreams were washed away?"
>
> Tracy43

It saddens me that when your ability to conceive has been taken away,
it is not talked about by any of the doctors or other health profession-
als that you deal with while going through this terrible disease. In my
situation,* I was left to deal with it on my own without anyone mentioning the situation.

While I completely agree that my health and survival is of utmost
importance, I still consider the other quality of life issues of equal
value. I was expected to just be thankful that my cancer was stabi-
lized for the time being, but how can I fully appreciate that when at
the same time all my dreams were washed away? How are you supposed to feel when you go from a vibrant young woman with her entire life ahead of her to one that has limitations, poor prognosis, and
infertility? Confused, dizzy, numb . . . . .

doowop

*Doowop was first diagnosed at the age of twenty-five and was in remis-
sion for four months before her cancer metastasized to Stage IV.*

I, too, am dealing with infertility. I just found out in April. I really wanted to have a baby (I'm not at all interested in a career) and it's amazingly difficult to have all that washed away. Frankly, I'm more sad about that than I was about the cancer. I'm sure that sounds strange, but for me, it was easier to deal with the idea of not having a life than it is to deal with the idea of having a life without purpose.

I know, I know, everybody says I can find another purpose, but I have to tell you, it just doesn't seem that way from where I sit. I'm going to counseling to try to sort it out, but I'm not hopeful that it'll solve the problem. I just keep looking at all these family heirlooms I take care of so carefully, for my future and now nonexistent children, and imagining them all in the inevitable flea market.

I couldn't deal with everybody's platitudes about it, so I went to see my 93-year-old grandmother. She's been through it all, and she very calmly said, "They're trying to be helpful, but they don't know. It's a disaster. There's no use pretending that it's not. It's an absolute disaster, and you just have to face it head on. My advice is to force yourself to face it and talk to yourself about it for as long as it takes. Talk out loud if you need to; talk to someone else if you need to, but talk to yourself about it until you're done. You'll cry a lot, but if you don't face it head on, and you try to ignore it, it'll cause trouble for you later on." I'm doing my best.

alleeum

I have grieved through most of the not-having-my-own-baby thing. I wish I could adopt, though, or at least foster a child. In my current situation, I am Stage IV and on chemo indefinitely, so having anyone under my care and responsibility is preposterous. It's harder now that I am about to turn 30 and my peers are flowing through all of these milestones. It is by far harder than any of my surgeries and initial diagnosis. But I will forever enjoy all of my 11 nieces and nephews, who I cannot spoil enough!

doowop

I guess I have been in the denial phase of grief over never having a child. I work with lots of women that complain about their children and how I should be glad that I "can go home and do whatever I want." My family all put on a brave face and none of them can stand my tears, so for them I am the funny and brave little soldier!

    KatRDH

Doowop and KatRDH,

Reading your e-mails makes my eyes fill up, but at the same time, I'm so grateful to hear from somebody else in the same situation. I know what you mean. It's hard when absolutely everyone else around you seems to be having babies right now. My stepsister and I had both independently decided to start trying to get pregnant at the same time, and we joked about racing to see who would get pregnant first. I got diagnosed, and a few months later, she started without me.

KatRDH, I, too, have told the people around me. Frankly, I just don't want to be in any more of those "when you have kids" conversations, trying to fake it, so I'm hoping to preempt at least some of them. It's hard enough . . .

Doowop, I feel for you when you say you can't adopt or have foster children. I really think that's going to be my situation, too. I continue to try to think of ways to make a mark on the next generation, to do something good in the world. I'd like to think that's what wanting to have kids is mostly about, anyway. (And so far, I've managed to get myself about 65 percent convinced.)

    alleeum

I was pregnant at my diagnosis and all opinions were to terminate. All I ever wanted was to be a mother. I had/have no "career" aspirations. I am fulfilled being a mother. It is very hard for me to see a mother or father with several children. I remind myself that some women can't bear any children, so I am very blessed to have one. He is 3½ and a pretty spectacular kid. At this point, I don't want to do anything that might jeopardize my health and risk my availability to him after what he went through this past year. But I still avoid baby environments. I haven't had a period for more than a year. I've experienced hot flashes. I am 37.

Helen

HAVING CHILDREN POST-TREATMENT

I absolutely want more children, but that's all on hold right now as my oncologist wants me to wait until I'm two years post-treatment. I was diagnosed with breast cancer about 18 months after my twin daughters were born, and to this day wonder if there's any connection between being pregnant (needed to use medicine to conceive due to polycystic ovaries) and having breast cancer. Consequently, I go back and forth about having another child. I have two beautiful girls who are happy and healthy, so why risk my health? On the other hand, I absolutely love being a mom—it brings me so much joy, happiness, and pride—so why not grow a loving family??

Alicia

> "I am living proof that miracles can happen."
>
> nam

Having a surrogate

For me, not having children has been the hardest part of this "breast cancer." I was only married one month prior to diagnosis. I saw a fertility specialist that put me on Lupron in order to shut my ovaries down. They were hoping it would avoid that area during chemo, but I was on high-dose (experimental) chemo, so it didn't work. Later, my very smart oncologist told me that I was not advised to get pregnant anyway, as I was ER positive. She said she allowed me to shut the ovaries quicker as it would possibly help me, and she didn't want me to lose hope of having children, so never told me until after I was in remission that I could never get pregnant. She suggested surrogacy for me, but I didn't have the time to save my eggs, so we are actually fortunate enough to have found a wonderful woman who is now going to be our surrogate, the traditional way, using her own eggs and my husband's sperm. We are hoping to have a family by next year. This has helped me in going on with my life, and although it was very hard to accept in the beginning, now at least I don't worry that I may pass this horrible disease on to my offspring. However, I did not have to give up on my dream to have a family.

surviving soul

SOLOMONIC CHOICES: WEIGHING MATTERS OF YOUR HEALTH OR HAVING A BABY

Because I never went into chemically induced menopause, my ability to have children never changed. My attitude about having another child, however, did.

Prior to breast cancer, I had a son and a daughter who were almost five years old and 18 months old at the time. Before my diagnosis, my husband and I seriously considered having more children, at least one and possibly two more. From a moral standpoint I just felt it would not be right to bring another child into our family if there was a chance that I was not going to be here to care for it. Yes, I know, none of us is guaranteed tomorrow, and that includes people who've not been diagnosed with cancer, but when you are slapped in the face with your own mortality, you understand the fragility of life.

When I was first in remission, I really had a problem when friends were pregnant, and as my children get older, I still have problems with baby showers and such because it is painful. Perhaps it will get easier when I am out of my childbearing years, because it is always in the back of my mind.

DawnMarie

I had become used to the idea of not having another child. I was diagnosed last January. I have had fertility problems all my life till finally I got pregnant with my now 7-year-old daughter. I have always wanted more kids and I don't feel fulfilled not having any more. My most concern is the future of my child. I wonder if I had another child would that jeopardize my life and rob my child of a mother. I can't take that chance. I need to be there every step of my child's life as I can. I dream and always hold a newborn with tears. I want so much to have another.

chemoangelbon

Chemoangelbon,

You can always adopt. This is what I did. It is not an easy road, but it will not alter your health. And you get to hold a newborn; it is your own. I never realized what a big part cancer had in stopping a woman from having children until I got breast cancer.

pinkwings

My husband and I got married when I was in my early 30s. We were about to start a family when I was diagnosed 4 years ago. After my chemo was over my period came back and my doctor put me in medical menopause. I am still in menopause and really want children. Because of my age I need to make a decision soon. In a way it is almost more cruel to physically be able to have children but not know what the effect on me will be. Nobody knows what will happen and this decision weighs on me daily.

Kim W

My friends have never been sick and are having kids and have no idea the daily internal struggle that I have. My problem is that I want a

100 percent assurance that pregnancy won't cause a recurrence. Obviously I will never get that assurance so I must use all of the information that I have and follow my heart.

Kim W

I had two girls after breast cancer. I waited two years after my last treatment and got pregnant very quickly. The first pregnancy was planned and the second was a surprise. Two healthy, happy baby girls later I am living proof that miracles can happen. At the same time, I will not have any more. I feel that my body has been through so much and I definitely had a fear that all those surging hormones might impact my chances of a recurrence. It is a hard thing, thinking you might not be able to have children when you want them.

nam

I was 30 when diagnosed and told that I may never have children due to the effects of chemo. This was one of the hardest things I had to accept on top of the fact I was being thrown into a complete out-of-control spin. Well, three years later I was blessed with a baby boy, born on Christmas Day nonetheless! (To me that is God's way of answering my prayers.)

Survivor Chick

MISCARRIAGE . . . A ROUND-ROBIN OF EXCHANGES AMONG THE WOMEN

"I am *so* tired of calling all my close family and friends with bad news."

Francesca

I had found out that I was pregnant in April; it was a surprise and I was not expecting to have more kids. Well, I had a miscarriage this weekend. I was 12 weeks pregnant and the baby just stopped living. I had to have a D&C and am devastated. I was not even sure that I was ready for another baby, although of course I would have loved it and welcomed it as I did my other two planned children. I was worried about the fact that it might cause me to get sick again, or maybe take me away from the other two. But now that is moot. And I am *mad*. I don't want anything else taken away from me: my health, my baby, my peace of mind. I am *so* tired of calling all my close family and friends with bad news. I feel like a burden again. I am 34 and my OB/GYN says to try again if I want. Do I want? The baby was probably genetically deformed. In other words, I did not cause it with too much soda, picking up the other kids, etc. But did all that radiation affect my eggs? Does God have another plan for me?

Francesca

Francesca,

I, too, lost my baby. But I had to make the choice to terminate to receive the best treatment for me, to be here for the child I already had. During the procedure I developed an infection and was hospitalized for four days. I felt like I was being punished for making that choice. I can't bear to be around mothers with children the age mine would be. I miscarried before this pregnancy. It is all devastating. It hurts so much. But know this, you did nothing! Perhaps God's plan for you is that you won't get sick again and you will be here for your children.

You are in my thoughts and prayers,

Helen

I am also sorry to hear of your loss. I also suffered a miscarriage prior to breast cancer. It was a very hard time, but this too shall pass, as they say. I'm glad to know that we have this outlet here for whatever our needs are. Each one of us here can relate, to some degree, and you should know that you are not alone, nor are you to be pitied, but there are ears to listen.

surviving soul

I can totally relate to you. I was trying to get pregnant before my diagnosis. I got pregnant on my own at age 36, but then miscarried at 7 weeks. Then, I couldn't get pregnant for 10 months. So I went the in vitro route. I became pregnant with triplets (2 embryos were implanted and one split into identical twins). This was quite a miracle. They all had heartbeats at about 7 weeks and then died a week later. I was diagnosed with breast cancer several months later. Needless to say, it was such a traumatic year. I thought infertility was the worst problem in the world, then I got slammed with cancer. But, in a strange way, the breast cancer gave me some sort of relief, a reprieve from trying to get pregnant. I *know* I will have a baby, one way or the other. I just try to look at all of this as an opportunity to grow and learn.

Lesanne

Thank you everyone. I am less angry today, although I am still really sad. I am the person everyone looks at with pity. I do not want to be that lady. I am too independent and strong for that. So, I am grateful for this chance to share with you all, who understand loss and grief so well. Your words have helped me tremendously.

Francesca

FOR THOSE OF YOU WITHOUT CHILDREN

Have any of you without children experienced this? More than one survivor acquaintance of mine has said that women with children fight harder to live. Now what kind of statement is that? I understand all of you with kids certainly have different worries than those of us without. But I think we all fight pretty damn hard to live.

My husband and I decided not to pursue fertility treatment or adoption after my cancer. Partly because we are both genetically challenged (me with BRCA1, him with polycystic kidney disease), and partly because we enjoy and appreciate our life together the way it is now. We were two weeks away from in vitro treatment when I was diagnosed. So it's not like we were not planning to have kids. Breast cancer made us sit back and appreciate what we have, not what we don't. Remaining childless has its benefits too. We laugh about it after a nice long weekend with the nieces and nephews after we spoil them and send them home!

Captiva96

Captiva96,

That stinks that someone would imply you need a child to fight this crap. I do have a child, and love her dearly. But I now wonder if she will get breast cancer. Or if seeing me suffer has scarred her. Or will she be motherless sooner than later. I wouldn't have it any other way, but I always tell my childless friends/couples go see movies, linger over your meals, have sex during the day, take off unfettered now because once you have a child you always need to consider them before you do things. You fight this because you desire to live. Enjoy the life you have. You have your priorities right.

Mamaper

Thanks, we do appreciate our life with no complaints. I was 10 when my mom had breast cancer the first time, 15 the second. So living with my risk was always there. It was in 1978 and people still kept this disease very hush-hush. My parents thought they were helping by hiding much of her pain and suffering. Now I realize that talking about it more instead of brushing it under the table may have helped me understand my own feelings at diagnosis. Even though I almost expected to get it someday, the reality of BRCA1 still hit me hard.

Captiva96

WORRYING ABOUT RISK OF BREAST CANCER FOR YOUR DAUGHTERS

Being a carrier of the breast cancer gene, I am very concerned for my 23-year-old daughter. I have had many discussions with my surgeon and oncologist, but the fear for her is stronger than the fear I have of my breast cancer being metastasized.

smilie

> "I am a firm believer that knowledge is power and I have tried to give my girls as much power as possible!"
>
> sgsmiles4u

Dear smilie,

My 33-year-old daughter and I are also BRCA carriers. I too am more concerned about my daughter and her young daughters than I am for myself. My daughter's reaction was to try to hide her fear from me, but in truth she was panicked and depressed. She elected to have a hysterectomy which has put her into menopause. I am despondent over this. Now she's talking about having a bilateral mastectomy with reconstruction. I am also concerned about how this will affect her future relationship with her wonderfully supportive husband. On the other hand, she and her husband say they are willing to do this to try to prevent any cancer from occurring. I'm more optimistic as I think in the near future far less barbaric options will open up. So far, though I give my opinion (I can't help it!), I try to be vocally support-ive of her decisions. I'm proud of her, as she has been so proactive, even starting a group for other BRCA carriers in her town. As much as this thing has brought us closer, I hate that I have passed on this genetic mutation to her and pray that her daughters have escaped it.

Juneboomer

Dear smilie,

I too have a 20-year-old daughter; I don't know if I am a carrier or not. I guess I should ask. My mother and my mother's sister both had breast cancer; my aunt succumbed to it at the age of 49. It was a bit scary when I was diagnosed. My doctor told my sister that she was at a much higher risk for the cancer than my daughter, but I really need to ask. The thought of "passing" on this trait to my daughter is truly scary. Juneboomer, you have a very brave daughter. My daughter has also mentioned just not having kids and having a hysterectomy, I couldn't believe it and was stunned, but I guess it must be incredibly frightening for our daughters and sisters.

ally

It is scary to know that possibly you have passed on a gene that will interrupt the lives of your daughters (and possibly sons; yes, men get breast cancer too) but cancer is no different than any other illness. I have actually passed on bipolar disorder to my child. We have to let go of the guilt though because this was not our decision to make. If you had known, would you have chosen to miss out on the joy of your children? Maybe, but probably not. We can only inform and educate our children about what is going on, let them make the decisions they make, and support whatever decisions they choose whether we agree with them or not.

zoochild

I hope being so honest and open with my daughter has made the thoughts of having cancer not as scary as when I was diagnosed. My mother died from breast cancer 5 years after diagnosis, so I thought breast cancer meant death. Here it is, 14 years survival, and I couldn't be healthier except for the normal aging process. Having discussed options with my medical team, we decided the best plan of action would be for my daughter to get a baseline mammogram at age 25 and to start seeing a breast surgeon on a yearly basis. If anything did occur it would be caught early.

smilie

Daughters! I have a 22- and 18-year-old and it concerns me daily. Their strongest ally is *knowing* that their father is diabetic and their mother carries a genetic dilemma that has caused the women in their family to have breast cancer! I did the genetic testing, but do not carry the BRCA gene. I was, however, the 9th member of my family to have breast cancer and once I found that out, I had a bilateral mastectomy rather than just one. I am a firm believer that knowledge is power and I have tried to give my girls as much power as possible!

    sgsmiles4u

We have a very strong family history—maternal grandmother, maternal aunt, my mother, and now me, and God forbid, our daughter. But interestingly, she is not afraid as much as she is wanting to learn as much as she can to understand what lifestyle choices she needs to make to reduce her risks, and hoping that with research, she'll not have to follow the path I have gone down. I hope that I have been a good role model.

    Big Red

My daughter is just about to turn 18. I have not discussed her risk profile for breast cancer with her but I did make sure she mentioned it to her doctor at her physical last week. I am worried. I'm not trying to avoid it but I think I'm just trying to get myself centered on what this means for me for the rest of my life. I do admit that one of the first things I thought of after diagnosis was what it meant for my daughter, especially since she already has had to deal with severe chronic asthma and many life-threatening food allergies for all her life—she doesn't need another thing to deal with!

    stellaluna

Stellaluna,

    I too had allergies, asthma, and spent a couple of bouts in the hospital growing up. I also *always* knew that my grandmother died of breast cancer. My mom was always upfront about staying on top of breast health because of that. It wasn't too much for me. As a matter of fact, it may have saved my life. I knew from an early age that regular checkups, self-exams, and mammograms were imperative. Thankfully, it was a mammogram that found my cancer, hopefully early enough to cure me.

CarynRose

KEEPING A JOURNAL AS A LEGACY FOR YOUR CHILDREN

I often think of doing some type of a message to my kids. I hate the thought of leaving them behind. I think it would be much easier if they were older and on their own. But then I think there will always be some reason I would want to stay around (at least until I'm too old to care). What are some of your ideas for messages? Videotape, letters, journals, scrapbooks?

ally

> "I want to leave something of myself to my grandchildren so they will know me as more than a branch on the family tree."
>
> scrapper

My children are grown and leaving them was still my biggest concern. When my mom and dad died my children were very young. I realized that not only did I lose my parents, but my children lost their grandparents. They had their grandparents on their father's side, but they never got to experience family life on my side of the family. My parents were wonderful, interesting, and talented people and my children don't even remember them.

Yes, having a plan is a great idea. But it doesn't apply only to those with young children who need to make provisions for their care. It applies to all of us. Writing a journal would be a way to let our children and grandchildren get to know us as people should death come for us too soon. Rather than being a mysterious face in a photograph, or the subject of a story told by another relative, we could reveal ourselves as living, breathing human beings with thoughts and feelings and attitudes. I want to leave something of myself to my grandchildren so they will know me as more than a branch on the family tree.

    scrapper

I adopted my son when he was 6 weeks old. When I was diagnosed my son was 11. I sat down and wrote a 21-page letter to him to tell him all my thoughts and to tell him the story about his family. I agonized over what I should tell him about his birth parents and that he has two brothers, one older and one younger, or how to go about finding them if he chose to. He has known he was adopted from an early age. Well, I did put all the information in the letter that he would need, and I think it made me feel better. You would be surprised at some of the things you can think of to write. My son will be 19 this year; I have added 23 more pages to the letter over the last 7 years and will continue to add to it. Maybe someday it will be as big as a book, but I will have covered everything I wanted to say to him. It was a way that I could look back on my life and make the right choices in the future.

    Jackjoy

My boys were both teenagers when I was diagnosed—one was away in college, the other in high school. I didn't make tapes or write letters but I think that is a great idea. I did talk to them often about what was going on, not just about being sick but about life and how much I loved them. We became much closer than ever before. I wanted them to learn how to face adversity and the pain that life often brings, whether it's cancer or divorce or any other challenge in our lives. In a way, I wanted them to learn how to go on living their lives and not fall to pieces or become very bitter. I wanted them to learn that you always have hope and faith and love and that even if I lost this battle that nothing would ever separate us, not time, not space, and not even death. I would always be with them in their memories and hearts.

Eve

WORRYING THAT YOU WON'T BE AROUND TO SEE YOUR CHILDREN GROW UP

My greatest fear—my children and their welfare. I want them to be well cared for and I want very much to raise them to adulthood, share in their successes, see them have their own families . . . all those things. The thought that I may not was the most terrifying thing in all of what I faced. I also realized we need to have a plan, and a good plan, for our children in case anything should happen to both of us.

junebug

> "In the face of death, only love has meaning."
>
> Eve

I feel so badly for you younger gals. You have a whole bunch of extra stuff to think about that those of us who have grown children don't have to think about. But that said, I would urge any and all of you, if you don't have a will, get one drawn up. I tell this to everyone. Whether they are battling breast cancer or in perfect health. See a lawyer and a financial planner. Get your duckies in a row. If you live to be 95, it won't have hurt a thing. If you don't, you could leave problems that would be handled by a will. It's not something any of us want to deal with but if we are wise we will deal.

Nett

I am afraid for my daughter. You see, her father had what turned out to be a terminal illness. And she and I lost him. She was 8 years old at the time, and he had actually lived longer than they said he would. We all know how much little girls love their daddies. So I wonder how she will handle it if/when something happens to me. At least she is an adult now, married, and has her hubby there to help. We have not been as close as I would have liked and that *is* my fault. I want time now to get closer to her, and my granddaughter also. But I am scared that she will not want to be closer to me in fear of the pain of losing me like she did her dad.

    SacredHeart

All three of my kids responded in totally unexpected ways. For the most part, it has brought me and 2 of the children much closer together. I worry about my oldest because she and her father aren't speaking, and she and her sister don't speak, so if something happens to me she will be very much alone, as far as family goes. For me death wasn't a concern, but leaving my kids was a major issue.

    kathi1964

PART THREE

The Big Picture

CHAPTER ELEVEN

Anniversaries and Milestones

"I try to celebrate the anniversary every day
with kind words to my family and myself."

Helen

W*e tend to think of anniversaries as moments for celebration, and some women are able to look upon the date of a diagnosis or surgery as something positive because it means they are here—alive and doing their best to be healthy. As one woman writes, "we know what is important now." Birthdays or wedding anniversaries become doubly happy moments, sometimes shared with family and friends, and sometimes spent as a day to be pampered, alone and by choice. Just as valid are those women who actively choose to ignore these markers, finding that it's important to have life seem as normal as possible, although to a woman with breast cancer* normal *is never* ordinary. *Even that gloomy national date, 9/11, receives comment here as a marker for a more profound loss of innocence. But perhaps the most poignant comments are from women who are young, under the age of forty. Their honesty—and their tears—are deeply moving.*

"The dates of my diagnosis and surgery will never be forgotten, but when the actual day comes around I do not 'go back there.' Going back to a bad thing that I can't change makes me feel helpless and pitiful and I just won't go there."

Noel

"I celebrate my anniversary with a spa day."

Lauren

"I used to hate to tell people how old I am—not anymore! I'm excited to reach each year."

webfoot45

"TODAY IS THE THIRD ANNIVERSARY OF MY DIAGNOSIS"

Today is the third anniversary of my diagnosis and the day before my 48th birthday, and I have been living with cancer now for three years. I don't know whether to laugh and sing, or cry! But I am certainly planning to eat my yummy birthday treat (old family favorite, icebox cake, anyone else ever tried it??) tomorrow, however I feel. Two pieces!

I know when I hit 50 (and five years surviving!) I will have a huge celebration with my family and all my best friends from everywhere who can come. But it will be turning 50 that I am celebrating, not dwelling on the cancer.

On the other hand, when I hit anniversaries of lost loved ones (my in-laws, my former minister who was like a second dad to me)

I cry for a good part of those days. I have been to three funerals since my diagnosis, and I find them very hard. What to do? I usually end up making a donation in the person's name to a charity; that helps a bit.

songbird

Dear songbird,

First of all, Happy Birthday!

I think that for me, each anniversary of something is individual. Some years I handle them better than others—the sad/upsetting ones that is. June 28th is the five-year anniversary of my surgery. I think I was more scared as I was being wheeled into the operating room than I'd ever been before, so remembering the day is both sad and happy. Sad because it was literally the end of my life as I knew it, and happy because I came out of the surgery alive and recovered. Then of course there are the happy anniversaries: marriage to my husband (going on 11 years!!), birth of my dear daughter.

There are lots of moments in my life that I wish I could forget. Like the one that comes up each year on the day my 15-year-old friend was struck and killed by a drunk driver, or the day that a lifelong friend died from AIDS. But the one I haven't yet begun to deal with is the anniversary of my 45th birthday. September 11, 2001. I think it will haunt me the rest of my life.

abrenner

Abrenner,

I know what you mean about September 11th, especially as I work in Washington, D.C., and I had to walk 8 miles home that day, seeing the smoke billowing up from the Pentagon, and being scared to death about both the terrorism and my own situation (I had just received my bone mets diagnosis the week before and was scheduled for a CT scan on 9/11). I had not told most of my colleagues yet about the mets, and it was very hard to walk slowly home (took us three hours) with five other colleagues, not mentioning both the pain in my back and my absolute fear that my kids were going to get attacked also. I have never cried so hard as that night at dinner, having gathered our family safely home, when I thought about all those kids in New York and Washington who would not be eating dinner with their moms and/or dads ever again. I was positive my kids would soon have this experience too. Thank goodness I was able to move on from that moment after much help.

songbird

The dates of my diagnosis and surgery will never be forgotten, but when the actual day comes around I do not "go back there." Maybe it's a coping mechanism, maybe I instinctively refuse to relive sad things because I don't want to be drawn into thinking about what I could have done differently. Abrenner and songbird, your experiences with September 11 are indeed haunting. Celebrate survival. Have another slice of icebox cake.

Noel

WHEN YOU'RE UNDER FORTY, ANNIVERSARIES AND BIRTHDAYS ARE UNIQUELY EMOTIONAL

Today is my birthday, and I have felt very emotional today, like I just want to cry all day. I remember feeling this way last year on my birthday. Now I think this year the feeling is heightened by going to the visitation tonight of the child that lives across the street who died of cancer Saturday. But I feel like I am so blessed to be here, and so happy to be here, and I know that had I not found the cancer I might not be here. I can't explain it to anyone, because it leads me to want to say, you don't understand. Because they don't. The only ones who can understand are those of us who have been thru this ordeal. Does any-one know the feeling I am speaking of?

pinkribbongirl

My birthday is this week—I will be 35! Someone asked me if I was sad to be 35, the beginning of a new demographic and sort of the start of middle life. I said, *"Hell no,* I'm not sad! I am thrilled to turn 35! And 40 and 50 and 90!" But I do not feel like celebrating my birthday either. What I would really like for my birthday is to spend the day by myself and be thinking about everything. Instead I am going to an amusement park with my kids and a neighbor and her kids. I'll ride the real roller coasters, instead of the emotional ones.

Francesca

Anniversaries are hard, even when I am unaware. Last Monday was my sister's 40th birthday. We had a wonderful day. That evening I went into a depressive state. I found it hard to get out of bed and cried for two days straight. I finally came to grips that my biggest fear is not making it to 40 myself. Talking about it openly and writing is very therapeutic for me. All of your notes help as well. Your honesty and courage inspire me and teach me that I am not alone in my feelings. To my fellow survivors . . . . *thank you!*

Mindymit

Mindymit helped to start a support group for women with breast cancer under the age of forty.

Young women talk about diagnosis, treatment, and survival as anniversary markers

Today is the one-year anniversary of the day I found out I had cancer. It has been a difficult day emotionally. Did you find that you had a hard time on anniversaries of diagnosis/treatment starts/treatment

ends? I have a lot more to go—my other surgeries, my radiation, my
end of treatment, etc. etc.

    Francesca

Francesca,

    Last week was my one-year anniversary also. What I underesti-
mated was how strong my emotions were toward the day and also
the worry of the one-year mammogram. My treatment finished 3
months before and I felt so relieved—thank goodness it's over! Then
it dawned on me that it wasn't over. Last week for me was emotionally draining and I hope as the time goes by I can relax at this time
a bit more.

    Meta

Francesca,

    Anniversaries will always be very emotional days, so I try to view
them with a different spin. I use them as a time to celebrate that I am
still alive. I have two anniversaries I celebrate—the day I found the
cancer (February 14 of all days) and the day my recurrence was discovered (October 10). My family knows that these are my days, and
we celebrate them somewhat like birthdays. We have a special meal
together and do something fun. The fact of the matter is that I will
never be the same person I was before the cancer (nor will they) so it
really is a *birthday* in a sense. Some of the changes are definitely bad
(no kidding!), but some are good too, and that's what I choose to acknowledge on those days. Congrats on your anniversary. You've survived a very difficult year. May you have many, many more
anniversaries ahead of you.

    happytobehere

I celebrate my anniversary with a spa day. My hubby knows that
January 18th is my day. He takes care of our son and I go to get pam-

pered. I really look forward to it and I am so relaxed that I don't think about the cancer anymore.

Lauren

I wasn't really thinking about the anniversary of my diagnosis until I realized I was being very difficult, an unpleasant person to be with, both for my in-laws that I was living with at the time while undergoing radiation treatment and my poor little three-year-old, who was away from home, friends, and his daddy. Then it dawned on me: it is March 4th, the day I received my diagnosis, and March 7th, the day of my surgery. This kicks off a difficult anniversary *month* for me, ending (but not really) on April 2nd, the day we terminated the pregnancy of our second child. At the July 4th festivities and parade, I couldn't bear to acknowledge families out with their babies, even though I'm so blessed to have this great little guy. So every day is an anniversary of sorts. I try to focus on the great stuff in my life and not dwell on the bad. I try to celebrate the anniversary every day with kind words to my family and myself.

I like Lauren's idea of a spa day. But which day I'll pick? End of chemo, first clean PET scan, day of diagnosis? I'll have to think about that. Or maybe just each day treat myself to something special, even if it is just my daily meditative walk.

Helen

I go with the day I was diagnosed, on November 4th. I decided to do that since that is what Lance Armstrong does, and I think he happens to be pretty cool. My husband and I have decided we will celebrate that day by going out to dinner, though I love Lauren's idea of a spa day! I was very emotional on that day last year, which was my first anniversary.

pinkribbongirl

After going through a metastasis I no longer think about my "anniversaries." I am just grateful to be cancer-free and have a second chance to live my life. But I sometimes still suffer from "survivor guilt" as it were. That feeling of why am I still here while others have been taken by this dreadful disease. There is no answer or reason, so I just try to live and appreciate my life.

    panthergirl

I've had my doctor and therapist tell me that I should do something for myself to *honor* my journey, yearly survival, and such. It seems weird to do something positive to honor this insane "battle" (that feels more right to me than using "journey").

    shari

I love parties, celebrations, and entertaining. This past year, my five-year anniversary was in October and my 40th birthday was in September. So I combined the two and threw myself a great big party, drank, danced all night and celebrated my life. All those that I invited and that attended were those that shared in my journey (family, friends, neighbors, and coworkers). I had just as many people at my celebration as I did when I went through this terrible ordeal the first time. I agree with your doctor that you should "honor" not just your journey, but your success in "where and who" you have become through your journey.

    Krista

I make a "thanksgiving dinner" to thank G-d for being with me throughout this ordeal and for having healed me. When I mentioned to someone recently that I have to start planning the next one she asked why I make one every year; my response was that I'm thrilled to make it and I hope to be able to continue to do so for many more years to come!

    miri

"ENJOY EACH DAY AS IT COMES . . ."

When I remember my anniversary of diagnosis it just is re-traumatizing and not helpful. It can even cause me to have panic attacks. So I just go on with my life and if I happen to remember how many years it is (two) I am happy and grateful to be here. But I don't honor the anniversary, I just continue my life as it was, which is always trying to be in the moment and enjoy each day as it comes.

pineapplejoey

I don't celebrate cancer anniversaries. I feel a little like pineapplejoey, that anniversary is one of trauma for me, not joy. I do, though, make much more of a big deal about my birthdays. I used to try to hide them, but now I make sure everyone knows. It is a celebration of my survivorship (isn't everyone's birthday?) and also of what I consider one of the biggest gifts of this crappy experience, that I'm so much less focused on my age, and what I "should" have accomplished. I used to hate to tell people how old I am—not anymore! I'm excited to reach each year.

webfoot45

CHAPTER TWELVE

Mortality

"I keep reminding myself that my soul cannot
be boxed up, and that helps."

Mawsquaw

Mortality is pretty much like the elephant in the room—everybody knows it's there but hardly anybody speaks of it. I would bet even the woman who's told she has a precancerous condition thinks about mortality. Frankly, it's unavoidable, so the question is how do we deal with this? How far do we allow our thinking to go in this direction? How would you want to be remembered? Are considerations of mortality different if you're under forty, or if you're dealing with an aggressive, potentially fatal, cancer?

The only time I seriously worried about dying was not long after I was diagnosed the first time, in 1990. It was evening, I was overwhelmed, and zoom—I went to that horrible place called "what if." "What if I die?" I asked aloud. My fear seemed to suck the air right out of the room. But then something wonderful happened. I remembered being a girl and jumping into a pool and letting myself slowly sink to the bottom; once there, I would push off with all my force and come soaring to the surface. And that's when I had an epiphany: I knew I would be fine, and with that knowledge came the realization *that whenever I hit bottom I will always bring myself back to the top. If you've ever been a swimmer, you develop a feel for how long you can stay underwater before you need more air; you learn how to survive, and that's what I experienced. In that moment I learned how to live.*

> "Don't spend your waking hours worrying about when you're going to die."
>
> MoxieAir

DON'T STOP THINKING ABOUT TOMORROW

I found dwelling on what might happen just brought me down. I could still be hit by a bus tomorrow and be out of here! This perspective has gotten me through some really rough patches. It has also given me reason to live today, right now in this moment as full as I am able. I am doing lots of stuff I was saving for later. For me, right now is later.

Picassa

> "Live each day to the fullest and with integrity."
>
> MoxieAir

The first thing I could think of is I am going to die. Then I thought of my boys and grandsons and my husband. I cried for a spell and then I pulled myself up by the bootstraps and started making plans for my treatment. I couldn't help but think of things that I wanted people in my family and my friends to have when I was gone. I started to go ahead and start giving things away, and then I thought, stop this nonsense! I thought, I am going to live a long time and I am not going to give up. It was a rollercoaster ride for me for a while, but I finally leveled out and started thinking clearly. Now I just take it one day at a time.

DollyD

> "For me, right now is later."
>
> Picassa

Each of us are individuals, and we handle things differently. For me, the worrying has stopped as my cancer has already metastasized *but* is being kept at bay for the time being. I have made peace with myself the past few months and am now trying to make peace with others in my life. For me, life has not returned to normal. But then, what is normal??? The way it was before breast cancer? Life always changes. My life could have turned out this way even though I did not have cancer.

The other night, my grandson and I were playing "Go Fish." It intrigued me, first of all that he knew how to play this game. But secondly, that the idea of "Go Fish" is relevant to us. Think about it. Don't have a match? Go fish. Don't have a "plus" for the day? Try again tomorrow or somewhere else (go fish). It is a weird analogy, but I hope that you see what I am trying to say.

Ladyblue930

> "I know I will be here tomorrow and so I set out
> to do my best each day."
>
> Grace

LIFE IS NOT A DRESS REHEARSAL

Are you a worrier? Or are you someone who looks forward to all your tomorrows?

"I often ask myself how long I will live"

Sorry to start a morbid line of thinking but it's one that pops into my mind frequently. I have looked for studies and asked my doctor about rate of survival for someone with my cancer and treatment but I don't think anyone really knows because the treatments I (we) received are so very different from those in the past. I often ask myself how long I will live and I keep getting an answer of six years from my little inner voice. (Yes, it's a strange thing to do but I've learned that I should check in with my little inner voice and balance it with what my head tells me.) I was wondering if others have thought about their personal longevity and what conclusion you've made about how you live your life today.

PattyS

It's a crapshoot, PattyS. Any two gals, with the exact same diagnosis and treatments, can die at hugely differing times out. It's not about when we die; it's about how we have lived. Don't spend your waking hours worrying about when you're going to die. You'll think you've finally figured it out and then *bam*, you get hit by the proverbial truck. Live each day to the fullest and with integrity.

MoxieAir

I have a 2-year-old son and it frightens me that I may not see him grow up. I have felt compelled to discuss my wishes with my husband regarding if things didn't work out in my favor and it is so hard because we are both only 38. A year ago it would be inconceivable to me to discuss my final wishes with him in detail because we had our whole lives in front of us. Cancer changes everything and there are no guarantees. I think it is our responsibility to make every day count.

AuburnLiz

I think we have all faced this question in one form or another. How can you help but look ahead and wonder if you will be here next year or five years or fifty. All I know is that I will be here tomorrow and so I set out to do my best each day. If we think about death too much we forget about life and it is the quality of life, not the quantity that matters. This said, I think it might be easier for me because I do not have young children. I cannot begin to imagine what that must be like.

Grace

What is that saying—life is not a dress rehearsal? I wonder also. Cancer is a very scary word and thing. MoxieAir has the right idea I guess—live life to the fullest and do what you can.

allegory

I think everyone who has faced a life-threatening illness like we have thinks about death. I think it's natural. I don't think it's healthy to dwell on it though. None of us know exactly when we are going to die but we know it's going to happen sometime.

The other day someone from the Canadian Cancer Society phoned to see if I still needed a volunteer driver. The woman and I started to talk and I have no sweet clue how it happened but she told me she had MS and is now in a wheelchair full-time. She knows she is slowly going to get worse and worse, but she was so positive, so full of life. How can I complain when there are others out there facing far worse situations? All in all I'm healthy, can get around, can still work, love and play.

Fun Lover

BE HERE NOW

Dying was never on my agenda. When I was diagnosed I did what I had to do. The protocol was surgery with nothing else. My second diagnosis of bone mets two years later was the same thing. Dying never entered my mind. Who knows, maybe I was in denial and maybe it's just my personality. All I know is I read everything I could but seemed to only retain the positive info. It was as though I didn't think all that negative stuff could apply to me. I recently found out that when I had the mets I had less than a 2 percent survival rate. Who knows, maybe I was in denial and maybe I'm just so ornery that the disease shriveled up and died.

hotflash

> "Dying was never on my agenda."
>
> hotflash

I was 38 at my diagnosis and as a former Vegas showgirl/professional dancer and athlete, I couldn't figure for the life of me why I got cancer. I have never had a fear of death for many reasons. One: I believe that God has a plan for me and I am divinely guided through the good and bad. Two: my father and many family members as well as all my favorite kitties are up there waiting on me and finally, the big reason is because I know why I was born (to get cancer and start a non-profit for breast reconstruction) and that gives me strength to go on. I *never* think about death or will I get it again, why me, or any of these things. They are not *living in the moment*—they rob you of doing just that by creating worry and negative energy.

MyHopeChest

In 2003 she began the website myhopechest.org.

WHEN RECURRENCE TRIGGERS
THE "M" WORD . . .

There is a cliché that the first thing a person thinks when they hear they have cancer is "I'm going to die." I didn't. In fact, it was probably a good two weeks or more after the diagnosis, when I'd already had my lumpectomy and was getting ready to meet with the medical oncologist and radiation oncologist, that I suddenly thought, "You know, this could kill me . . . I could die from this!" I have a vivid recollection of that moment, standing in my kitchen. And I burst into tears.

Up to that point, I had been very focused on surgery options, understanding my pathology reports, treatment options, tests, etc. I was getting lots of information and making decisions. Since then, I don't think about it much. I do worry about recurrence (not obsessively, but it's there), but I don't really worry about dying from cancer. Of course, when someone I know passes away from cancer, that makes it more scary and makes the possibility seem more real, but I don't think about it too much.

kamaha

> "I use to worry about recurrence. I now pray more and leave my life in God's hand."
>
> twinsmom

I think about dying fairly often. One does that when one has had a recurrence 9½ years after the initial diagnosis—a metastasis from the original breast cancer of almost 10 years ago! Considering all I've been through, I'm doing well and back at work half time for now. All scans, MRIs, and blood tests are, for the moment, clean. I really thought it was out of the woods. I know I will never again be so complacent!

BarbS

I think more about dying now (after breast cancer) than when I was diagnosed. When I was diagnosed, I was angry. I was ready to fight that demon. I thought more about death while sitting in the chair for my first chemo treatment, reading the release form. Then it hit me. The treatment is worse than the disease! I could die! Exactly what were they putting in my veins? I didn't have a clue, but I was willing to give it a try to save my life. I feel so awful, I'm still wondering about death. I never did before. When will these feelings, emotions stop?

Blessed

For those of you who are more than 5 years out, does the worrying about breast cancer ever end? Do you ever stop thinking that any new ache or ailment is a metastasis? Does life ever completely return to normal?

Raesinthesun

Raesinthesun,

I do not consciously worry all the time about a recurrence or metastasis, but the fact that this could occur is always tucked away in the back of my mind. I feel that I must try to control the breast cancer and every situation as if it were a job no one will do for me. For me, easing off on control can be difficult.

Flower

I didn't really think about dying until after my second lumpectomy. I had a reaction to the morphine and stopped breathing. Man, what a jolt that was. However, I did regain my perspective when I got home from the hospital, so don't dwell on it much. A friend I used to work with died in November from her colon cancer and no one told me. They thought it would be too negative as I was beginning chemo then. When I found out in December I was shocked (sad for her and her husband) and really went into a funk for a few days. Then I picked up myself and went on again. I guess we do have lots of those ups and downs with this disease, but I don't think I'll ever be complacent, just too many possible scenarios. I just pray that I'll die at 90 of something unrelated to cancer (I'm 56 now)!

RedBird

Living with multiple recurrences: in support of Gtown mom

I also didn't think of dying really at all initially, except for one day. I went in for my pre-op chest X-ray and got a call asking me to come back the next day for another X-ray. They said that something was on the X-ray, and it was probably a shadow from one of my ribs but they wanted to make sure. So for 24 hours I was a mess, thinking that if the cancer had already spread to my lungs, I was dead. Thankfully, it was a shadow, and everything was fine. My oncologist said that I could consider myself cured, since 75 percent of women with my type and stage of cancer never have recurrences. I liked that and didn't think about recurrence. That was in 2002. I had my recurrence one year after my initial diagnosis. Since my recurrence and multiple recurrences in the chest wall and the fact that all of the different chemos that have been tried have not worked well (until this current combination), I have thought about dying on and off. I try to not think about this, as I feel that it is counterproductive to my trying to get into remission.

I know that my future is uncertain, but I am aiming for 3 years, when my son graduates from high school. From there I will aim for another 3 years. My oldest daughter will probably get engaged this summer and I *need* to live to walk down the aisle with her and see her happily settled. I go to counseling every week or two and that is about the only time that I "open the door" and think about dying, about the "what ifs." I cry and then close "the door" and move on with my life. As I sit here and type this, I am teary. I can't think or talk about this without the tears and the emotions.

Gtown mom

Gtown mom,

I am so sorry you have had to endure so much. I guess if we had to "get" something, at least we got an illness that is subject to a lot of research and receives tremendous funding. On another note, I have relatives who have had cancer diagnoses with poor prognoses. They have beaten the odds. The statistics are just numbers and are not certain for everyone. I think your decision to aim for three years is a good one. Enjoy this time as much as possible. And, as the end of the three years draws near, plan another three! You may need to do more planning than you thought.

Ellen

Therapy as an aid and a guide

I was diagnosed in 2001. I had a lumpectomy, axial dissection, chemo and radiation, now on tamoxifen. So far things are looking good. But I did and still do think of dying too much for my liking. At first I took a lot of Ambien for 2 years because I couldn't shut my eyes at night without thinking horrible thoughts, but now I am sleeping pill–free. I can't say I have exactly come to terms with it, but I think it's more like me and my shadow . . . or me 'n my mortality? It's always there to a degree. I just try not to let it rule my life. But I still wake up crying sometimes when I think of my world going on without me in it. I know I need to find a way to get beyond this. Am considering therapy, which I never had before.

Nushka

My thoughts about dying and recurrence became easier to deal with when I shared them with my counselor. She helped me put some of the fears to rest, be realistic about the "what ifs" and begin to look forward. I can share stuff with her I would never say to my children or my close friends. She helped me through grief periods for my husband and parents' deaths, so we've been through a lot of ups and downs. Helped make me get calmer and helped me get off antidepressants.

RedBird

WHEN SOMEONE YOU KNOW DIES FROM BREAST CANCER

"It was a defining moment for me and different than any other death I'd experienced."

bradleyteach

I don't want this to be a morbid topic but I was wondering how all of you feel when someone you know with breast cancer dies. I just came back from a funeral of a young mother who died of breast cancer unexpectedly. Besides feeling her death and pain for her children and husband, it scared *me* terribly for myself. I think that I could accept it for myself but I kept putting my children and husband and family in the place of my friend's family who died. I had to have a conversation with my family about me dying because it scared all of them too. Believe me, this is *not* the conversation that you plan to have with your children at 42. This woman was my age and had "talked" me through my cancer 2 years ago as she had just gone through it before me and had done so well. Pretty scary. I will just keep living every day without regret and to the fullest. This just reaffirms it. You ladies are the only ones who will understand this.

    newday

During my treatment last year, someone who I became acquainted with as a result of my diagnosis passed away from her breast cancer. She had lived with recurrent metastases for several years and when I first spoke with her, I'd never have guessed that in six months she'd be gone. She wasn't someone that I knew very well or was close with but her death came as a horrible blow to me. This person's experiences had been so valuable to me in facing my own cancer. It hadn't occurred to me how deeply I'd be affected by the passing of someone from the disease that I was currently fighting. It was a defining moment for me and different than any other death I'd experienced.

    bradleyteach

Newday and Bradleyteach,

    I too lost a friend to breast cancer shortly after I was diagnosed; our sons were the same age. It shook me terribly. Soon after that we began losing members of our local support group (all ages), including one who I found truly inspiring with a real zest for living. After that I stopped reading the obituaries. It was too painful because I found I knew more and more of those with breast cancer.

I also lost my youngest sister to breast cancer last year. She had bone mets at diagnosis and seemed to be doing okay. It all came up so suddenly from vision problems in October to her death in March. It was not only terrible to lose someone so close, but leaves me and my family wondering "what if" and my sister's family wondering "why us." A breast cancer death is certainly different from all others, especially a young one.

lambda77

About 2 years after my diagnosis, I stopped by our only hospital to visit a young woman with advanced breast cancer. I was very sad when she died a short time later. I stopped by the mortuary to pay my respects when one of the employees of the mortuary asked after my health (knowing of my breast cancer). I tried to tell him I was doing well, but couldn't—I was overcome with tears and had to leave. How could I tell him I was fine, when someone was dead from the same disease?

asp

While struggling through my roughest moments of chemo, an infusion nurse introduced me to this marvelous creature who was struggling with the same protocol as I, the major difference being that the doctors were trying to manage her cancer, not cure it. Her breast cancer (same stage as mine) was not treated aggressively enough when first diagnosed and it had metastasized to her liver. She got me through the roughest times and we commiserated like only those of us who belong to this fucking club can. Her husband called me tonight to let me know she died yesterday (Sunday). I talked to her only last Tuesday. When I hadn't had any return calls to the several messages I left I knew something was up. I am so sad and so scared and so angry.

Sad because I didn't have enough time with her. Scared because although I am good at denial, I can't deny that what they say they cut out of me can kill me (will kill me?). Angry that our health care system let her down, not only when she was originally diagnosed and as recently as last week when the nurse didn't urge her to come in when her abdomen was as swollen as a 6-month pregnancy. Lastly, I guess I am determined. This woman had lost her best friend to breast cancer less than a year ago. I want to survive this so that her husband, family, and friends can know a survivor, so my family and friends can know a survivor. Cancer cannot be allowed to win.

Mamaper

Death among members of your support group

Today I found out about the death of another lady with breast cancer. This makes 4 women this week that I've been acquainted with. I am sick to death of this damned disease. I am tired of being scared that it's going to take me next. You group with others that have breast cancer for the support, but what is the support when they start dropping like flies? How do you get comfort when the people that used to comfort you start dying? This whole support group stuff is a double-edged sword: when it's good, it's good, but when it's bad it doesn't get much worse!

kimmytoo

I understand this all being a double-edged sword. There is *no one* that knows what we are going through except other survivors so that is who we naturally turn to for support. For us right now there is nothing worse than them dying of the disease we live with and fight every day. After my original diagnosis I did not go to support groups for the very reason that you talked about. If I went for support and then they died I think it might have been worse.

Kim W

> "How do you get comfort when the people that used to comfort you start dying?"
>
> kimmytoo

I am active in an online support group and board. We will be 4 years old this month. We have lost 2 members in that time, but the other day, we lost a 3rd, and not to this stupid disease, but to a car accident and that has shook up everyone even more. She had finished treatment, good prognosis, and now this.

It does make you really look and see in your life what is important, what really matters. To try and do what makes you happy, gives you satisfaction in life. To tell those around you what they mean to you. Live each day to the fullest you can, don't waste a day. I don't mean live as if it's the last day you will have, but cherish each one that you have.

jealta

TOO YOUNG TO DIE

> "I miss the feeling of being immortal that I think most people feel in their 30s, even though we know we aren't."
>
> pinkwings

I was 35 when diagnosed and 36 when I finished treatment. Just after I finished treatment I had a very vivid dream that I was in the hospital dying and my son was crying over me. My husband was crying and facing out the window. I think about dying every day.

I read somewhere that surviving cancer is like stepping off the curb and getting hit by the proverbial bus—surviving, but never being able to get back on the curb because you are forced to stand there in the street waiting to get hit by the bus again.

   Max's Mommy

> "I no longer fear death the way I did before,
> since I've been forced to face it head on."
>
>   surviving soul

I miss the feeling of being immortal that I think most people feel in their 30s, even though we know we aren't. I never let things bother me before, but now every headache must be a brain tumor, the aches in my bones must be from bone mets, etc. It is hard to live like this, and I miss my more carefree life before breast cancer.

   pinkwings

I agree with you, pinkwings. I sometimes envy others who don't even consider their mortality. The only consolation for me now is that I no longer fear death the way I did before, since I've been forced to face it head on. I also plan better then I did before, and really do try to enjoy the little things. I look at life through the same eyes, but in a very different way.

   surviving soul

> "We aren't supposed to be contemplating our
> mortality when we are this young. It's just
> wrong."
>
>   LukesMom

WORRYING ABOUT YOUR CHILDREN

> "My daughter needs me and I need to be here for her."
>
> Still Here

I really wish I could say this wasn't an issue for me, but it's a huge issue for me. I live 3,000 miles from any family and I'm a mom of 2 teenagers. When it comes to guardians of the kids I really struggle as I do not want my children uprooted and brought somewhere they will have to learn to adjust to after their parents are gone. I think it's our responsibility as parents to make arrangements in case anything happens to both parents and yet as of now I really feel between a rock and a hard place. I really have no one near me that I feel could be a good guardian for my children so I pray daily that if one of us has to go please don't make it both parents before the kids are old enough to be on their own. We have made sure that financially they would be taken care of for a very long time. But it would never replace parents. Sounds crazy, but after cancer I take nothing for granted anymore. Anything can happen and it usually will so I worry; my son will be 17 in 5 months so I have 1 yr and 5 months and then I can stop worrying. Crazy, huh?

Princess86

Nothing like taking the bull by the horns. When I was first diagnosed with breast cancer, I was angry and scared and sad but I didn't in my core think I would die because of it. When I got my BRCA1 diagnosis I started to wonder if maybe I would. When I got my leukemia diagnosis I kind of figured well, hell, there go my already slim chances of living a "normal" lifespan. Not to say that I have given up! But two cancer diagnoses kind of make one wonder.

I can't say I've made any peace with any of this. I have an

overriding imperative desire to live in order to be here for my 2¹/₂-year-old daughter and my husband. That is what truly keeps me going and moving forward. My daughter needs me and I need to be here for her.

That being said, cancer and the possibility of early death are the elephants in the corner, always present on the periphery. The question I keep coming back to is, "How do I want to live my life?" The answer that keeps returning is "I want to really *live*." I want to really live and be present in my own life, not a bystander wondering about what-ifs and might-have-beens. Easier said than done but I try.

Still Here

I used to think that if I died tomorrow that I have led a very fulfilling life. Then I had my son and now I would like to make it to 100. When I was pregnant and diagnosed with breast cancer, I just wanted to make it to see what my baby looked like. Now that he is almost 2, I just want him to know what I look like.

Lauren

> "I fear the disease less than the thought of what it will do to those I love when I die."
>
> songbird

I think about death and it scares me. I honestly believe that God has a special assignment for me. I am divorced now, and was presented with the idea of a will needing to be made. When I think about whom I want the twins to live with, I just freeze up and go on to something else. The twins are 3¹/₂ now. I want to see them graduate from college and my grandchildren. I know this is something that I need to address, but maybe in time.

twinsmom

"It's not a case of being afraid of death. It's a case of being sad to leave those we love."

Mawsquaw

I am like many others, most scared of leaving my family behind. My children are still young. I fear the disease less than the thought of what it will do to those I love when I die. I pray every day for strength and courage for myself, and also for them since they may have to grow up faster than most kids if something happens to me.

songbird

THE "LITTLE BLACK CLOUD"—EVEN WHEN THE FORECAST CALLS FOR SUN AND BLUE SKIES, SOMETIMES IT'S HARD NOT TO CARRY AN UMBRELLA

I now realize that I have always been afraid of a premature death, so getting cancer to me just confirmed my worst fears. Although my prognosis is quite good, not an hour goes by where I don't think about it. I tend to fear the worst. When I asked the docs about what the chances were I wouldn't beat this, they said about 20 to 30 percent. Unfortunately, I focus far too much time on the 20 to 30 percent and not enough time on the 70 to 80 percent.

I am sure you have all heard someone say "I could die in a car accident tomorrow." These things are all true, but it does not compare at all to living with cancer on a daily basis. I call it my "little black cloud," always over my head casting a little shadow over me, never letting me quite forget or completely let go.

Alix

For me this is the worst part of cancer—the mental games I play with myself. The surgery/treatment I was mentally prepared for. I've always had a "gotta do what you gotta do" attitude when it comes to medical treatment. I was invincible before my diagnosis. Now death is a reality.

I'm sure, like most of you, my cancer does not match anyone else's. I don't fit into any of the risk groups. So it makes me question every well-meant reassuring word. I think that is hard for "outsiders" to understand. They tell me I have the best prognosis. But they were also the ones that were surprised I had cancer in the first place. Cancer has destroyed my positive, optimistic outlook on my health. I want that restored!

> D'sMom

Fear is such a small word for what we feel. You wonder what you'll miss, if you will be missed. I don't have children, but I have many children in my life. I wonder about the events in their life I wouldn't be there for. Then the sky opens and everything is blue, and I realize that I can no more control the outcome of breast cancer than I can the weather.

> DianaRmn

LEAVING LETTERS TO TELL YOUR STORY

I may not be able to join up for the next three days (due to a little 20th anniversary trip!) so wanted to get this out in the open before I forget to ask. Have any of you written letters or made videos with messages from you to your children/spouse/friends etc., in case you die? This may seem an uncomfortable thing to ask, but I am seriously thinking of writing such letters to my husband and kids (I don't think I could stay composed long enough to make a video) and wonder how I will feel doing it, and what I would really want to say. I think I have to do this. I am tearing up just thinking about putting words to paper that someone will read after I'm gone, but it seems so important.

> songbird

I lost a good friend who was also in my support group. At her memorial service the letters she wrote to her two children were the most meaningful and moving of the entire service. It is something they will have with them always. That she was able to do this only made us all more appreciative of what a terrific friend and mother she was.

    playwright

I've thought a lot about this and I'm still on the fence. On the one hand, the idea of leaving some sort of written or video legacy for my daughter and her children appeals to me. But I'm not ready to look at myself in terms of checking out yet. That isn't to say that I don't have a good will, and clear instructions to my husband and siblings about what I want in case I am in the position of being unable to make my own medical decisions.

I support and encourage anyone who wants to do this to go ahead, by all means. I've even suggested it to several people I've met along the way who've chosen to end their treatments. But other than creating memories for my daughter that I consciously "create" (such as our family vacations, letting her lead one of our Passover Seders this year), I am just not ready to do more in terms of leaving a legacy. She *is* my legacy. And I guess I'm probably in some denial, but I can't bear the idea of leaving her yet.

    abrenner

PLANNING YOUR FUNERAL

I have a perfectly healthy friend who wrote letters to her children, sealed to be opened upon her death. She urged me to do it but I have not; don't know why.

    betty

I think your idea of a letter is great. Ever since I was diagnosed I've been creating in my mind a folder with plans for my funeral. (And I fully expect to live, but just facing death gives one pause.) When I hear music that I would like for my funeral I think about what instruments would be needed to do it. I hate sad music at funerals, and want joyous music at mine. At the end I want the Hallelujah Chorus with everyone standing. This is to be followed by a great dinner, compliments of me, where people tell stories and celebrate my life. And thanks to your idea, I can add my letter to be read.

  Noel

I'm so glad to hear that others are thinking about their funerals, too. Being metastatic means mine is definite, though I'm certainly not booking a date! I think many people want things to be a certain way (some don't care, I suppose), and I take every chance possible to assume a little control over this whole process, since I have no real control over the progression of the disease. So, sure, music, speakers, format—I'm writing it all down. I think it will help those left behind. I know my parents really helped me by leaving something similar when they died.

  Daisy

Thanks, everyone, you all have such good thoughts to share! I have not written my letters yet, but we have updated our wills/living wills/powers of attorney recently, and I also wrote an essay about my life since college for a 25th reunion yearbook, in which I dealt fairly lightly with the cancer but still noted it and made sure to include some positive thoughts, such as what makes me happy and what I dream for the future. I gave this to my parents and they loved it. I have also recently made lists of all the things I love (from Vermont lakes to eggplant), things I don't like (from rude people to blue cheese) and things I believe in, which I hope my family will appreciate later. I am also beginning a journal of basic family history and traditions with my husband, one for each child, to include such things as where our ancestors came from (not a full genealogy, but a start if they want to look further), what we do for holidays, places we love to go, poems and writings I like, etc. It is sort of a memory book/scrapbook but without all the fussy trappings. Maybe I will be able to deal with the more personal letters to each child soon—I hope so.

songbird

Songbird died a year after this was written.

I had a baby 2½ years after diagnosis, which was a joyous yet anxious time for me. What if the cancer returned? What if I died before she really knew me?! Since my husband and I share a love of history, I began scrapbooking and immediately saw the powerful impact. My scrapbooks tell the whole story, and really let my family know about me. Starting this led me to teaching scrapbooking, and I'm so pleased each time I see another family touched by the love and history that pours into a book.

I also began writing letters to my daughter. Each month on her birth anniversary day, I'd sit down and write her a long letter, telling her about me, about her, and how very much she is loved and wanted. I kept that up for the first two years of her life, and then trailed off to occasional letters, when something is worth sitting down and pouring my heart out about. Writing is how I feel confident that I'm communicating to my family.

Janet

I am currently writing a letter to my post-cancer baby who will be turning 1 this Saturday. For his birthday, I am not having a standard party. I want everyone who comes to write him a card, poem, letter, send a pic . . . and how they felt when they heard he was coming and how the last year has been. I'm sure many people will discuss my cancer with him. All the stuff will be put away until he is 18, and God willing, I'll be reading all of it with him!

BCWarrior

CHAPTER THIRTEEN

When You Look in the Mirror, What Do You See?

"When I look in the mirror I see every other woman who has gone through this."

KellykO1

*M*irror, mirror on the wall, who's the fairest of them all?" I *can't begin to count how often I recited those lines when I was a little girl. Between Disney's Snow White and Cinderella, and Mattel's Barbie, it's a wonder I didn't become the queen of botox. If anything, I've gone the other way: rich moisturizer for the face and good shampoo for the hair are the mainstays of my toilette. As my friends and I often remark, one of the joys in getting older is becoming less vain and more comfortable with who we are, what one of the women below describes as "a developing sense of acceptance."*

But—and this is a significant but—when it comes to looking in the mirror, really looking first at your body and then into your soul, the picture changes once you've had breast cancer. Of course the cruelest period is when you're going through chemo and you've lost your hair, and your skin is so dry that no amount of cream seems to do any good. Those are tough days. Nobody finds solace in the mirror then. Gradually, however, improvements become apparent, both physically and from within. I can recall times I'd look in the mirror and shake my head in disbelief: "Is this me?" It wasn't that I'd suddenly grown up so much as that I'd grown older, and I didn't know this person, didn't even know whether I liked her. Even today, some years since the height of my treatment, I can see the impact on my face and body—I know which marks (literal and otherwise) are from cancer. We all do. I can also say that the mirror is my laboratory, where I examine my soul by looking at my eyes, my posture, the slope and pitch of my shoulders. Confidence, acceptance, pride, vigilance, concern . . . these make up the composite of what I think of as "me" today.

This topic about looking into the mirror—about self-reflection literally and figuratively—is one of the most provocative. Each woman was asked the question, "When you look in the mirror, what do you see?" Not surprisingly, the thoughts expressed are some of the richest and most profound in the book. I began to notice that the nature of the comments varied considerably from those who were newly diagnosed to those who had been cancer-free for several years. For this reason, the entries are presented chronologically according to the amount of time since the contributor's diagnosis, in three major groupings: from the present up to two years; from two years up to that magical cutoff number, five years; and from five years on. This isn't meant to imply that a woman who's been well for a decade doesn't feel challenged by the mirror; she does, but her perceptions are materially different from the woman who's three months out and receiving chemotherapy.

Above all, I was struck by the general optimism and contentment expressed by the women, regardless of their medical condition or personal life. With very few exceptions, this is a bunch who celebrates living, with its natural ups and its downs. But make no mistake: any of these women would gladly have "skipped" this life lesson, as made plain by the woman who wrote, "When I look in the mirror I see a woman who hopes to have one day when she doesn't think about cancer."

"I love to place my hand over my heart where my breast has been removed and feel my heart beating."

Hummingbird

"When I look in the mirror I see a future."

Meta

"Love what you got because you can live without a breast. You cannot say the same for the human heart."

Hummingbird

"I don't know who I see. It doesn't look like me and it doesn't feel like me. It's like a stranger looking back at me and I am not at all sure that I want to know her at all."

kimbasa

"At 65 I tend to be one of the 'invisible ones' out there in the world. Unless I smile. Everyone reacts beautifully to smiles."

Annie Mac

"I see in the mirror a new day every day. The best day is *today*."

rainbow

"When I look in the mirror, I see the flat chest of my youth."

Kay

"The heck with the mirror!"

lily987654

FROM THE PRESENT TO 2 YEARS

I just see myself, the way I always have.
Cath
Cath had a double mastectomy based on family history.

I don't know who I see when I look in the mirror. Truth be told, I try not to look into the mirror—my face with very little hair or my whole body. I know that I am me. I know who the "old" me was. I was outgoing, I was funny, I was upbeat. I was a mother, a wife, a sister, a friend, a daughter, a niece, an aunt, a neighbor. I am not sure who I am now. I know I am a fighter. I know I am determined, I am hopeful, I am a survivor. My mom always described me to others as a "mover and a shaker, and once she makes up her mind, you better get the hell out of her way because she is determined and she will do it." I think that still applies. I just am not sure how to go about getting to know the "new" me. I think I like the new me. My sister-in-law compared her husband (who is in Iraq fighting in the war) and me: we are both fighting wars. I know that I am winning.
mommy of 1
Mommy of 1 was diagnosed at the age of thirty-four.

I still don't have much hair, so I don't know if it will be thicker, or curly. I do have enough to see that it's mostly gray, which I expected. I keep telling everyone I look like a demented elf, running around the house in my winter hats because my head's always cold! Or that

I look like the old anti-smoking ads, you know the one with the old men, mostly bald, their chests caved in and their bellies sticking out. We need a warped sense of humor to get through this!

What do I see when I look in the mirror? On the inside, a survivor, someone who's strong and independent, but willing to lean on a shoulder when it's offered. A woman who's had to make tough choices and live with the consequences. A mother who wants to survive for my children's sake but who isn't afraid to die.

kathi1964

Kathi1964 was thirty-nine when diagnosed.

When I look in the mirror, I see so many things that sometimes they won't all fit at once. I am early in the journey and the past 2 months make me feel as if I am living in a time warp. Some days dragged waiting for diagnoses and treatment plans and others flew by. I am currently undergoing chemo, hoping to shrink the very large node positive beast. No one can do battle for me but it gets me through each day to know that so many are with me, cheering me on to the final victory. I too see the tired warrior, but one blessed to have so many who care. I look forward to seeing the strong survivor in a few months; I know she is in there waiting for the end of the journey. She will be back.

Scottie

Every day is a blessing. My family is even more important to me now. I am not just existing. I am living!

Aruba

Aruba's mother died from breast cancer.

When I look in the mirror, I see the me that has grown so much and so quickly through this horrible ordeal. I see a young woman who has beaten so many things in her short life. I see a mother who would give her breath for her daughter. I see a daughter who longs for her mother to stop feeling guilty for me getting this and not her. I see a sister who won't stop pestering her sisters to get their mammograms. I also see sadness and fear. I see pain and anger. I see a young woman that has just started to *live* her life. I see a wall that when it breaks will let loose a flood of tears that will be hard to stop.

> kw4184

> *Kw4184 was only twenty-nine when diagnosed.*

I see a woman wanting to grab on to life and yet is scared of losing it, so I stand trying to figure out where to go from here.

> shari

I think I look strong, bald head and all.

> JoAnn

I see a funny-looking face with a head covered in mangy chemo fuzz, a strange new hair color, and my eyes peering out through my glasses, and a determination to reinvent myself as this breast cancer journey unfolds. I see a woman who needs to create a new way to make a living, for my landscape design and maintenance days are numbered—I am concerned about getting lymphedema and not having the stamina to make gardens anymore. I see fear and sadness around these issues, for serious gardening has been my life force for years. I see lots of question marks floating over this funny head!

> goldfinch

I want to be able to look in the mirror a year from now or 10 years from now and never forget this experience.

> rainbow

> *Rainbow was diagnosed two months shy of her fiftieth birthday.*

I have only finished chemo, not had surgery or radiation yet, even though I should have about two months ago. I'm still taken aback when I see my reflection. I used to have long hair. Now my hair is about a half-inch long, and I have these odd wrinkles under my chin that seem to be fading with time. My coloring is good, and there is plenty of hair, so I guess things will improve, but I still don't recognize that woman in the mirror.

soccermom

Soccermom was in her mid-forties when diagnosed with IBC.

I see a scared girl who wants her mommy to make it all go away. I am scared to die; I am not ready. I want to be old and see my kids have kids. I also see someone who never thought I could handle all of this but when I am asked how I do it I say one day at a time and when people say I could never go through all of this and make it I say yes you can, having children you have to. They are the most important things in my life.

april_4_us

April_4_us was just thirty when diagnosed.

Most days I see myself as a warrior doing battle. My half-moon lumpectomy scar reminds me of a marking or tattoo, more like an initiation symbol than the result of a wound. When I first look in the mirror in the morning, I barely recognize myself in my hairless image and I feel somewhat invisible. But every day I paint on my eyebrows, choose my hat, and courageously step out into the world, clearly visible as a woman living with cancer. I'm not trying to be a role model or an inspiration; I'm just trying not to lose more of my identity than I have to.

Towanda2

Sometimes I look in the mirror and ask, "Who is this person? Is this really me?" I then look closer at my face and into my eyes and remember "Yes, this is me, I am still the same person, I just look a little different than I used to." I remember when I was a kid my mom would tell us the old adage "Don't judge a book by its cover." I guess that is something I have to do—not judge myself by the way I look, but by who I am, what's inside. That's what matters.

Sometimes I look at myself and think "no wonder my husband and kids treat me the way they do. Look at me—I don't look very lovable." It must be weird for them. I can choose not to look at the mirror; they cannot choose, they must look at me just as I am, even if they don't like what they see.

ally

Ally's mother and aunt died from breast cancer.

Who do I see when I look in the mirror? It depends on what day it is and what time of day. If it's morning, before I get in the shower, I do my usual and look to see if the scars have changed overnight while I was sleeping. I know after lying down they always look better (no pressure on them), so I like looking at them in the morning. If it's at night, they look more red, more irritated, and I once again wonder if they will ever fade the way I would like them to. As far as who I am when I look at myself, I see two people. One, a scared, little girl who wonders about dying young. Two, a brave woman who still can't believe she has made it through all this still alive, hoping to live a full life with her husband and family. I like me even more now. I know what I can do. I know what I'm capable of. I know God has a purpose for my life, which hopefully means I'll be sticking around a while longer.

Squirrel

From Squirrel's bio: "I went from hearing about breast cancer victims to being one." She was thirty-two.

I don't look in the mirror often—I tend to avoid doing so—and I'm ashamed to say that the reason is that I have gained more weight than I find to be personally acceptable. I don't feel it's "me" in that mirror; I feel it's "that fat person." And I have never been thin, not since puberty. It's just that I am now the heaviest I have ever been in my life, and I don't even have chemo to blame. All I have to blame is my own maelstrom of emotions from going through a) losing my job (and the feelings that stirred up in me) and b) getting this disease, going through a phase of "I don't know what's going to happen to me, so for now I am going to eat whatever I want." I had no place else in my life in which to overindulge: not sex (I'm not the promiscuous type who would do it with just anyone!), not money (don't have enough), so what I gave myself free license in was food. And I'm still living with the aftermath. No, I'm not huge. I'm just way heavier than I want to be.

Anyway, I do have to look in the mirror when I go on interviews. Do I completely like what I see? No. When I wear control-top pantyhose, all the fat rolls get pushed up to my waist and they show under my suit jacket. I hate that. I hate thinking I either have to buy a new suit or wear non-control-tops to avoid that. At the same time, I realize I have to be as kind to myself now as I can, even if I'm facing what seems to be an insane amount of challenges—to find a new job, to find a new home. At least I am doing it this time with my family as a support base. I hope that will make it all easier. And I hope that once I am reestablished it will be easier to say, "I don't need all that food. I don't need to stuff my face till the cows come home."

Annemarie

Some mornings I get up moving slow and a feeling little down and some nights I cry before I fall asleep but when I get up and look in the mirror each day it helps me to remember where I've been and how far I've come. I only think about living; I don't think about dying (I've found that kind of thinking only makes *me* sick, really).

When I got divorced I thought that was the worst time in my life, but when I was diagnosed with breast cancer I realized that the divorce was a small task to deal with, so now post–breast cancer I feel like I can handle most things. At the end of the day when I look in the mirror I see a stronger happier grateful new me.

    river

I am more and more aware that breast cancer is a *part* of who I am, but not my entire identity. So when I look in the mirror, I see someone who has had a breast cancer diagnosis and addressed it, but that is not all I see. So my breasts do not "match" (they never really did), but otherwise I am essentially physically the same. Cancer put life into perspective. I was going through a spiritual quest when I got my diagnosis, so I now see a more centered person in my mirror. Of course I also see a person with a whole new set of questions.

    Lizzi

I see an alien. I see someone who has a ridiculous "haircut," a different color of hair, bloated, and scared to death. I can't relate this "me" to who I was. I can see the fear in my own eyes, and I can't figure out how to get past that. I just finished treatment, and maybe I'll get some self-confidence back eventually.

    kimmytoo

    Kimmytoo was thirty-one when diagnosed.

I see a woman ready to tackle my new "normal" life and move on beyond cancer. I have a lot to live for and a lot to do before I die, so don't have much time for sadness and pity.

    RedBird

    RedBird is in her early fifties and has grandchildren.

I see a woman who tries to control other people's lives when her life needs to be controlled. I see a woman who can be abused and used (emotionally), I see a woman who is afraid to let go of old baggage. I see a woman who knows that she is blessed in many ways yet feel that she doesn't deserve these blessings. I see a woman who is afraid to pray for anything because she already has been blessed with an early detection of breast cancer.

ladycmj2004

I see a pretty, vibrant young woman with beautiful breasts, despite the scars. I love my hair even though it is short (and I have never had short hair). I see beautiful skin. So many people have told me that I am glowing. I think that comes from the inside. I have grown spiritually by leaps and bounds. Sometimes I feel sad and angry, but I accept those feelings as natural and move on. Generally, I am proud. I have lifted myself up, and I have met so many other wonderful people who have lifted me as well. I know that I am stronger than I have ever been before, and this is the gift of breast cancer.

Lesanne

Lesanne was thirty-eight when diagnosed, and has since had a mastectomy and reconstruction.

I see a woman who has changed so much in a year. I don't fuss about makeup or hair anymore. I'd rather spend that time doing something else. I really see now that my true beauty has always come from within and not in the outer package (just like Mom always said). I only have one breast but that's okay, I don't really miss it.

PMOMMY

PMOMMY was thirty-eight when diagnosed and subsequently has had recurrences.

I think I look prettier than I could ever allow myself to feel or think I did. I think this is in large part due to my diet. People tell me my skin and eyes are clear. I'm also at a great weight, which is easily maintained with my whole foods diet and lots of walking. And now that I have hair and fingernails growing back, well, what more could a girl ask for.

I also see a big scar, one lonesome saggy boob, and a port-a-cath showing through my skin. And I see fear. And I see someone who is stronger than she ever believed she could be. I see someone who will grow old despite the statistics and doctors' opinions. I see someone who will be an inspiration to her son, husband, and others because she refused to back down. I think this is my gift to give to others.

I look at myself in the mirror and I think, how did this happen. And then I think, move on and make the most of it. It could be worse. You are here, feeling good. You have everything you need.

Helen

Helen was thirty-five when first diagnosed, and at the time had to terminate a pregnancy. Soon thereafter she had a recurrence and bone mets.

I still see me. The smile isn't as spontaneous. The eyes look a little haunted but it's me. I actually can look in the mirror at the lumpectomy site without a problem. Maybe that's because I am so convinced that it's just a matter of time before there is a recurrence, so I am watching carefully for changes.

Nett

Nett's mother had breast cancer.

I love to place my hand over my heart where my breast has been removed and feel my heart beating. I remember doing this same action when I was a little girl lying in bed. Love what you got because you can live without a breast. You cannot say the same for the human heart.

Hummingbird

When I look in the mirror I see me: hopeful, tired, aging, young, happy, sad. When I look in the mirror I see every other woman who has gone through this.

KellykO1

KellykO1 was in her mid-forties when diagnosed.

I am two people. In my mind's eye I am an energetic thirty-someone who has the whole world ahead of her. Then I pass a mirror and the real world floods in. I am jolted every time I see what a year of treatment has done, but only for a micro-second. What has been done "to me" has also been done "for me." The mirror reminds me that I am 68 but still functioning on all levels and very grateful for that. By nature I'm an optimist and so far nothing has changed that.

Anna Marie

I don't see me. I see ugly. I see fat. I see a bad short hairstyle (and I wore my hair short before). I see short eyelashes and faint eyebrows. I see someone tired, even after a good night's rest. I don't like to look in the mirror anymore.

Max's Mommy

I see a much older woman than I was a year ago. It used to be that no one could really guess my age, thanks to my father's genes. I don't think it's so hard to see me as 38 now. I have curly hair now, which has drastically changed my appearance, at least to me. And after 3 months, I'm still not used to the woman who looks back in the mirror. She is almost a stranger some days, and only somewhat familiar on other days.

judy

Judy found a lump when she was thirty-seven. In her bio, she writes: "I thought I knew what I was in for. I actually had no idea."

I never really see me anymore, at least who I used to see. That has really bothered me. It's like I had one of those "extreme makeovers"!!

It is hard for me to just accept so many changes that I did not choose, and have this "just be thankful" attitude that I'm told to have. Yes, I am thankful for my life—don't get me wrong, but to be totally honest I find myself purposely avoiding mirrors! When I read positive responses they tend to baffle me a bit. What exactly did I miss through this life-altering experience? But if what they say is true that mirrors don't lie, then I need a new mirror!

 Bren

I see my naked self, and still can't believe how drastically my body has changed. I see two 8-inch scars where my breasts once were, that I am now referring to as my "badge of courage." I wonder how long it will be before the scars become almost invisible. Every morning when I step out of the shower, my reflection stares back at me, and I don't believe it is me I am seeing. And yet I know inside I am still me, although a diminished me, who still feels shame at how my body looks now, and I'm working on that. I've been told by a cancer coach it took great courage to battle the cancer for yourself and your family, and there is nothing to be ashamed of.

 Big Red

 Big Red, who has a family history of breast cancer, was in her
 mid-thirties when diagnosed.

I cannot believe it's only been a year (this week!) since diagnosis. It seems a lifetime. It's so odd that the woman I see doesn't seem familiar and yet I can't really remember what I looked like before, either. In my eyes I see incredible strength and a developing sense of acceptance.

 Agent99

One year after diagnosis, mastectomy, one less breast, and chemo, I don't really feel different but I know that I am. I can honestly say that this has been one of the best years of my life. Not because I am alive but because I *feel* alive. And if I do go through this again, I will be strong, not because I'm some superwoman, but because I have no other choice. You do what you have to do.

Marsha O

I see an imperfect but strong woman with a good heart and I accept that. Before breast cancer I was always trying to be so perfect and I've just learned to accept who I am now and have learned to love me. It's the truth although it may sound a little "mushy." I see a confident woman who believes God has a reason for all of what's happening and I don't think He's ready for me just yet;-)

1Faith

When I look in the mirror I see a woman who is determined to beat this disease. I also see a woman that at times is unsure of herself. However, when I look into the eyes of a stranger much like I did this past weekend and hear of a fellow sister that has refused to fight this disease because doctors have said she only has XYZ to live it makes me mad. The one thing I have found when I look in the mirror is a woman that can help others to learn that doctors are practicing medicine and that there is always hope and new things coming out every day. I have seen and talked with women in all stages of this horrible disease and let me tell you this is one mantra that we should all share. We who are here are the best medicine for those who know not.

Mel

Because of a strong history of breast cancer in her family (her mother died sixteen years after being diagnosed at the age of thirty-three), Mel took an aggressive, proactive course of treatment.

I don't look in the mirror very often. I stand in front of a mirror to put on makeup and comb my hair, but I don't often *look*. On the rare occasions when I do, the person looking back isn't me, at least not the me I knew. An older woman looks back at me and the spark is missing from her eyes. She lost two years of her life and cannot get them back.

Depression was creeping in and keeping me from seeing myself.

This group [the online Web project] has helped me gain confidence and made me realize that I must take total control, and they have actually given me the energy to do it. So I am now starting to *look* in the mirror and make friends with the face staring back at me. The scars on my body aren't pretty, but no one is perfect. I think the scars on the inside, the ones that don't show up in the mirror, are the difficult ones to deal with.

Stillhealing

I see a woman grateful to still be here and alive and continuing on the journey. Bitter and angry to be facing ongoing life and death treatments and decisions, with a 100-yard stare occasionally looking back out of the mirror, but refusing to have a victim's mentality. Scared that death may still come knocking. Hopeful that the journey will continue into a long life well lived. Flat-chested and scarred but undeniably feminine. A mother, a wife, a sister, a daughter, myself.

Still Here

She has gone through a mastectomy, leukemia, and had an oophorectomy.

I am sometimes not happy with what I see. I have gained so much weight since treatment, 35 pounds. I see the same eyes and smile but sometimes wonder "who is that pudgy person in the mirror?" Oh well, God loves me no matter what and this body is only a temporary vessel until I am in heaven and *perfect*.

Suzanne

Today I went and stood in front of the mirror and really looked at myself. I am still there: under the short fuzz on my head and behind the glasses I now have to wear and the new teeth because I lost mine, it is me. A bit older, a lot grayer, more drawn in the face, but it is definitely me. I just stood there and started laughing and then I couldn't stop. My dear husband came in to see what was going on and he really didn't understand when I explained it was me in the mirror but I knew what I meant and I'm sure you do too. I just lost track of myself for a while.

kimbasa

When I look in the mirror, I miss my eyebrows! I miss the hair a little, too. (I've lost it twice! It had grown about 6 inches when we had to start the rough chemo again.) I miss my breast, when I think of it. (I usually forget it's not there.) I miss my strength and stamina. But I think I miss my waistline the most. But, you know what, I like my smile. I think I'm smiling more these days. And a smile can make a big difference to a person's appearance. I'm happier. I take things slower. I get less stressed out about the little things. I'm alive, spending more time with my kids. The heck with the mirror!

lily987654

Since her diagnosis at the age of 26, she has had a couple of recurrences.

I see a woman who has evolved. At first, I thought it was God's punishment for my own vanity. (Now how vain is that thought?) Realizing that I was not specifically chosen to suffer brought me to the conclusion that I could be the one to steer this experience for better or for worse. I was not given a sentence as much as I was given an opportunity to learn, to grow, to teach, to reach out, to love.

Do I see a woman with no breasts? Or a woman who knows she is still one hot mama and it was her personality all along that was the attraction? But who can look at the chest when it is the sparkle in the eyes that holds your attention. (Today all I saw was a woman who needs a haircut.)

JodieR

I have spent the last 20 months getting to really know me. Now when I look in the mirror I no longer see the long blond hair. I now see dark short curly hair and often think, "Who is that? I don't recognize her." But who I see is not about how I look, it is about who I see when I look into my own eyes. In my eyes I see someone with a lot of pain, not just from the experience of breast cancer, but from many life experiences. I see someone who is very angry, very sad, very scared, very confused, and very lonely; but I also see someone who is on a journey, who has much to learn, and who is a very eager student.

Alix

Alix, who was diagnosed when she was thirty-seven, wrote that she'd prefer to "crawl into a hole" rather than express her anger.

FROM TWO TO FIVE YEARS

I was 28 when this all started and now I am 30. I had a bilateral, chemo, and reconstruction with many revisions. I see someone who is wiser than her years. I see someone who stared death in the face and lived to tell about it. I see someone who carried her family throughout her ordeal because they needed her strength to deal with her health problems. I see someone who hurts every time she looks at her daughters and wonders if they too will become victims of this terrible disease. Most of all I see me—I am still the same me that I always was. I am a little older, a little heavier, a little bit tired but still me. I am still beautiful.

KerryMcD

My treatments started when I was 34, and I'm now 37. I had a bilateral, aggressive chemo, radiation, and reconstruction. When I look in the mirror, I see someone familiar, but she doesn't feel like me yet. She's fat and misshapen and tired and scarred, and her breasts are strange with seams and uneven, skin-toned "nipples" like something out of a science-fiction movie. I miss feeling like "me"—the old me—and I keep working to get things back to "normal." I wonder if, sooner or later, I'm going to have to realize that this *is* normal from now on, and that the early-thirties me isn't ever coming back.

I wonder if, instead of aging day by day, like everyone else, cancer people are pulled out of their life at diagnosis and dropped back in when they finish treatment. If we haven't noticed our ongoing aging because we've been sick and distracted, it's no wonder we're a little shocked by it.

alleeum

Alleeum was around thirty-five and wanting to start a family when she learned that she had become infertile due to the cancer treatments.

At the beach I noticed these little hermit crabs. First I noticed how ugly they were. Ugly little bugs in my opinion and then as I watched them I saw how they battle to the death for their shells and one of them loses the fight and it loses the shell. It was interesting to me how he didn't give up. He immediately went looking for another shell and he seemed frantic at one point looking for a new place to call his own and then I started feeling bad for this ugly little bug and when there wasn't a shell big enough I found a shell and dropped it in for him. I found myself at the beach with little children around me relating to this silly little crab.

I saw myself in this crab. I lost my shell in a battle and for the last few years I have been searching for a way to make this new body comfortable and struggling for a way to feel free, to call it mine again. Then through the support, love, comfort of others, I realized that someone dropped me in a new shell and I began to feel safe again and peaceful and hopeful. That crab wasn't content with losing; he had drive and determination and that is what I see in a cancer survivor. That is what I see in me.

I should have brought that little crab home that day but I was too cheap. It made my heart feel good though when I noticed that the little boy who was listening to me talk to this ugly little crab then talked his mommy into letting him have it. As I saw him walking down the boardwalk with "my" little crab I really felt so good, like both the crab and I got a second chance. We both fought a battle and won.

Princess86

Princess86 was diagnosed when she was thirty-six.

From a physical standpoint, I look in the mirror and I am so sad. I have had bilateral mastectomies and the scars are everywhere. I feel like I have been gutted like a deer. My surgeon was wonderful and she did everything right, it's just hard to look at the outcome. I always had large breasts, and I am not missing those. I am a person who never let my breasts define who I was, so losing them was not the hardest issue I faced. But I think the total loss has affected my self-image more than I realized. I am anxious to have reconstructive surgery because I want so much to have something in the place where my breasts used to be. I know they won't be perfect and I am very realistic about my expectations, but I want something there.

tootie

I am so proud of the woman I see. I have come so far. I used to be such a wimp, and I am so brave now. I know I can handle what comes my way. I like the way I look, and my new hair. I don't mind the scars on my breast, under my arm, or my bikini-line cut. I can honestly say I do not care what anyone says or thinks about the way I look when I go out. I am happy with how I look.

pinkribbongirl

Pinkribbongirl was diagnosed at the age of thirty.

I am not my body and I am not my cancer. I used to be ashamed of what I saw in the mirror, and I would cringe whenever I looked in a mirror. I had a real problem with self-hatred, and there was hardly a part of my body which I haven't at one time or another found fault with and hated. But now I am proud of what I see. Cancer has changed me irrevocably, but to me it is a wonderful change, and I am in the process of becoming the kind of person I always dreamed of being.

Susie

Susie was originally diagnosed with bone mets and has since had a recurrence and hysterectomy.

I do not like my body shape and size. My light blond hair is now a definite brown. I would highlight or dye it, but I don't want to add any chemicals to my body. It has gone through so much. It took a while for me to adjust to seeing a dark-haired person looking back at me in the mirror, especially when passing through a room and catching just a glimpse of myself. I can't walk very well and must use a scooter at school to get around. It is hard sometimes to accept the disabilities caused by the treatments.

My bathroom mirror sees frustration many times. I have gone through some depression because I didn't like what was looking back at me. The counseling has helped me to see who I am really. It is the real me inside who is beautiful and happy that matters. In today's society that is not always easy to accept. I would like to feel pretty on the outside again.

Many people say to me that I don't look like I have been really sick and are amazed at my ability to smile, laugh, and enjoy life. I don't always see that person because I am looking at the surface of me with brown hair, a different body shape that I don't like, and clothes that don't fit like they should. I will be glad when I find the whole me looking back with one pair of happy eyes.

Linda

I am not very happy when I look in the mirror. I see a stronger woman than I used to be, but when I look down at my left breast, I see a scarred mess. I want it to look like it was before cancer, but I know that will never happen. I try not to think that every pain or twitch means bad news.

Purplepassion

I see a woman who is very fun and funny. A woman with the same body shape as my mother. A woman who doesn't sweat the little things. A woman who is able to give support to others with breast cancer. A woman who is terrified of a recurrence of breast cancer. A woman who is still able to open her heart to others. A woman I'm starting to get to know and enjoy being.

mtn woman

Most days I see strength and pride but occasionally the battle scars win out. My breast cancer diagnosis was tough but, thank God, so was I.

Gram K

Gram K was diagnosed when she was fifty.

When I look in the mirror, I see a changed woman. One who has finally come out of her shell, and grown from the once-uncertain insecure little girl. If I look deeper at myself, I truly see someone who has defeated all odds. I also still see sadness. This sadness is not because I pity myself for what I have gone through with breast cancer, but because I pity myself for not having known the strength I had all along. I don't understand sometimes why it took such an awful disease to wake me up.

surviving soul

Surviving soul was diagnosed when she was thirty.

I see someone who's older, grayer, and with curlier hair than three years ago. Someone who's gained weight, and is hobbled by the physical after-effects of some pretty rugged treatment. But I also see someone who's kinder, gentler, more forgiving, and more cognizant of her behavior and how it affects others. Going forward, I want to see someone who's gotten past her physical problems, and is strong(er) and slim(mer) but who still has the same hair (I love my new hair!). I want to see into the soul of the person looking back at me, and believe that cancer has given her a second chance at life; a chance when I get to the end of my days to be able to say, "You helped make the world a better place. You helped people. You did the right thing."

capecodder

When I look in the mirror, I see a series of contrasts. I see eyes that cry, yet a face that has laughed more since diagnosis than at any time in the past ten years. I see a frightened child who has nevertheless learned to subsume panic under a blanket of strength. I am older in body yet younger in spirit. I see a giant scar on my chest and many threads of silver in my hair, along with a renewed sense of physical connection to the world. I see a daughter, wife, and mother determined to shelter her family from the worst fears of the night, while letting them comfort her with words, helping hands, and love. I see a strong, capable professional woman, able to succeed at her career in spite of ongoing chemo, multiple side effects, and lessened energy. I see both faltering and incredible determination. I see myself as part of a survival team that includes me, family, friends, doctors and nurses, medicines, work, charitable acts, and faith in God. I see a soul searching for strength and courage for the years ahead. I see myself scattered over my favorite place in the world, and also dancing at my daughter's wedding.

I see dark nights and beautiful sunny days. I see the seasons changing with a feeling of hope. I am a hawk, soaring over the world and brushing those I love with the wind from my wings. I see myself committed to making the world a better place, striving to help those in need of healing and succor. I see hurt and anger sometimes, but mostly cheer and good humor. I see *life*. I see myself, forever and always.

songbird

Songbird was diagnosed at the age of forty-five, with eventual recurrences and bone mets. She died in 2005.

I see a daughter, sister, wife, friend, but mostly I see a mother. Since I was pregnant at diagnosis, my son and I have a very special bond. We went through 3 surgeries together and he truly saved my life. I am proud to be called "Mommy."

Lauren

When I now look in the mirror, I am happy to not be seeing the little old man looking back at me (the one who seemed to take over my face and body while in chemo), but I do see an older version of myself.

Marcia

Marcia's older sister was diagnosed with breast cancer more than two decades ago.

My mirror now shows several parts to my reflection: my emotions (some I can see clearly, others are jumbled), my physical form (I'm mostly okay with it, but I've had almost 3 years to look at it and get used to it), and some internal and external scars (some healed, some not).

I've also given some thought to the times I actually do stand before the mirror: getting ready in the morning and again undressing for bed at night. I realized I look only at specific things: brushing the teeth, I look only at my mouth (did I leave toothpaste running out my mouth?); putting on eye makeup, I look only at my eyes (is the eye shadow too dark?); combing the hair I look only at the hair on top of my head (did I get that bald spot on top covered?). I don't look at the whole me very often at all. If I really force myself to look, I can see the whole body, breast scars and back scars and all, but the point is, I don't look at the whole body much at all.

Bach

It will soon be four years and very slowly I am starting to look like myself again—a bit older and much wiser and even better in some ways because I learned so much at an age when most people don't even think about issues like sickness and death.

Eve

When diagnosed, Eve was forty-five.

Soon after surgery and for a long time during chemo, every time I looked at myself (usually after a shower), I imagined I saw: deformity, someone who "isn't what she used to be," pudgy and misshapen, and a whole lot of psychic pain that probably added to the poor self-image (feeling scared for no particular reason). And I dressed in really dumpy clothing (didn't want any of my body to show).

Now it's 3 years later and I see a whole new lady when I look in the mirror. I rather like her. I take care of her (and she takes care of me). Yes, one breast (the treated one) is smaller than the other and yes, a few new pains. But I feel so much better than the feelings (and image) of 3 years ago, even if I'll never be the same (oblivious) person of 10 years ago. And I have to say, that when I look in the mirror, I *like* what I see: the person, the survivor with grace and spirit and spirituality.

earthtobabs

When I look in the mirror I see a pretty tough lady. I see a woman who really found out how much she is loved and appreciated. A woman who touches teenagers' lives in many special ways (not just teaching them French or Spanish). I see a mom who has 2 precious daughters who look up to me and hope that someday they will be as strong and driven as I am. I see a wife who's adored by her husband.

I see a sister who is respected and loved by her siblings. I see a loyal friend who has only a few but very loyal friends.

I also see a woman who lost her best feature: her hair. A woman who has lost her strength and that at times has to struggle to go up the stairs. A woman who is too embarrassed to get undressed in front of her adoring husband because her left breast is *deformed*!!! My husband always tells me that the look of the breast doesn't matter to him; well, it matters to me. I see a woman who has aches and pains in every inch of her body all the time. A woman who blanks out in the middle of a conversation to one of her closest friends because she just can't remember her name!! I know you will all understand these 2 very different people I see in the mirror.

graciela0107

Ironically, I am not nearly the worrier I used to be. How I wish I could have become this face in my mirror without the need to pass through the pain and struggle of cancer.

mountainmomma

At this point, cancer is not utmost on my mind. I think most who are aware that I've gone through this think of it as a speck, something in my past. In my mind, it is always there. It has colored who I am, not good, not bad, it just has. Cancer does not own me. I have moved on. I want to look in the mirror and have no regrets.

RC

I don't think I am vain but when I look in the mirror the person looking back is a very different me. I think I have aged tremendously in the face, but I guess all is okay. My husband still thinks I am beautiful; he just can't convince me.

Jonniemac

Looking back to when I was in the midst of treatments, I saw someone in physical and emotional pain. Today, four years later, I see me.

I am evolving from what I was and where I came from. Breast cancer changed me, just like getting married did, just like having children did, just like losing people close to me did. It was a life-changing event, and certainly a very scary one, but I am still me.

junebug

Junebug was forty when diagnosed.

When I look in the mirror, I see a fresh me. I see short-cropped hair that I would never have had the courage to cut, but that I enjoy spiking with gel as it grows in post-chemo. I was a bottle-blond; now I love the natural dark color of my hair, and how it complements my eyes. I see a dented breast through my snug T-shirt, but I don't care. I feel comfortable with my new body—heavier from tamoxifen, but healthier because of it. I see a woman who, at age 41, has gained wisdom beyond my years, but alternately has regained the youthful love of life and the joy of the moment. I now see how much I love life, love my family, love *me*, and how strong my fight is to grasp as much as I can possibly hold.

buckeyemom

Buckeyemom's mother died from breast cancer.

My bedroom closets have mirrored doors, together making an entire wall of mirrors. I try to avoid facing that direction when I open my eyes in the morning, remembering the day I stared at the gray-haired old lady lying in my bed. Feeling stronger after some coffee, I return to shower, dress, and do the best I can about my appearance.

I was never a great beauty, but have big, brown, deep-set eyes. Those are still the windows to my hopeful, life-loving soul. The anxiety I saw every day for nearly a year is almost gone now. My 61-year-old skin is not wrinkling much, but I have laugh lines that I kind of like. For a long time after surgery I skipped more than a split-second look at the two horizontal scars on my chest. Now they are just a reminder of my journey through terror. And my victory. I am thin and can clearly see the ribs behind the scars. When I strap on a mastectomy bra with pockets and silicone breasts, the effect is a near-return to my old chest. Except for *no cleavage*! The rest of me looks pretty much the same as before cancer; it's helpful to have some tethers to my old body for self-recognition.

auntann

People told me that I was so strong to go through what I did and that they could never do it. I feel that I am just stubborn, not necessarily strong. I was diagnosed with a very aggressive 3B and wasn't given much hope. I considered that a challenge. Oh, yeah, watch me. I am going to beat this thing. I am competitive and don't like to lose. I also think I am so wise for my 38 years and understand things that most people my age don't. And about my body I admit sometimes when I look in the mirror naked it is still a little strange not to see breasts. It has gotten easier over the years and I have come to accept the "new me" most of the time but sometimes I wish I was "normal." But as we all know, I am alive and that is what matters.

Kim W

When I look in the mirror I see: A wife, mother, daughter, friend, teacher, and mentor. I see a woman, who, although her body may not be perfect, her spirit is indomitable.

I see me, only better. I see a survivor.

DawnMarie

DawnMarie was thirty-four when diagnosed.

The mirror is not my friend because it shows only the outside. But if I look deeper into the mirror, past the face and the scars, I can look inside and see myself, and the picture is much different. I see a woman who thanks God for each and every day. I see a woman who yearns for a simpler life. I see a woman with a big heart and desire to help anyone or anything in need. I see one who loves tending a garden as much as tending her children and that dusting and cleaning toilets will always be there tomorrow.

lambda77

Lambda77 was thirty-five when diagnosed and is the oldest of four girls. One sister has died from breast cancer and another from ovarian cancer.

FIVE YEARS AGO AND BEYOND

I had chemo at age 39. Before chemo I was always getting compliments that I looked much younger than my age and I live in a college town with lots of beautiful young women. I always took pleasure in that. After chemo, my hair came back grayer. I also put on weight, and my skin is not as youthful looking. Now at age 43, no one ever says that I look younger than my age. I wonder if this is a normal part of the aging process, but in my heart I know the chemo aged me faster than what would have been normal for me.

On the brighter side, when I look in the mirror, I also see someone who is more knowledgeable about life. Having the experience of cancer has put me in the position of being able to help others. I like seeing this new side of me.

Tracy43

When I look in the mirror, I see my mother's daughter; a strong, determined, loving, compassionate, humorous, and courageous woman who is a survivor.

Autumn

I have always seemed to see only my flaws. Before the cancer, I would say I was a pretty normal looking person, except first thing in the morning! I was average in size, looked a little younger than my years, was pretty energetic, could work a 10-hour day and after a little rest, could maybe put in one more hour of work time. My body felt almost as young as my mind still did and that was at 50. Now I feel I look 10 or 20 years older than I am. After all the chemo my hair is just plain weird, the texture is wiry, and the color is a mixture of white, gray, and dark something. I used to have auburn, reddish-brown hair.

My body of course changed shape; it all slid downhill and I guess a pear is as close a description as I can get. To put it bluntly I look old and tired. Because of the bone mets I don't stand straight anymore and my energy level is, what energy—the 15 minutes when I first get up in the morning? So, gee, that is so depressing, but the upside now. I am still here with my daughter. I can still cook a meal and do some of the chores, even though it takes me a lot longer. I can still make people laugh and smile, and to me that is important.

NMRose

NMRose died in 2007, shortly before this book was published.

I am 60 years old and I like myself better today than I did 10 or 20 years ago. I just bought a really pretty lacy summery pj from Victoria's Secret. It is sexy and someone else might think I look so odd with my one breast and the other side flat. But I'm used to it and it was never ever an issue with my husband. He tells me I am his girl forever and I am!!! Even though I am angry at times that I have cancer, I am more at peace with myself as time goes by. I think it has something to do with realizing what the important things in life are . . . family, friends, and roses.

Sue

When I look in the mirror I don't recognize myself anymore. I can't put my finger on the exact reasons, because I still look a lot like I did before my cancer journey, but I don't *feel* like I did before my cancer journey in so many ways. Except for the physical attractiveness/sexy issues, I can honestly say that I really like who I see in the mirror. I'm still putting the pieces together to my "new" life, but so far I like where I am.

abrenner

Both her mother and grandmother survived breast cancer.

My mastectomy scar is only 5 weeks old. I had lived for 5 years with minimum scarring after my lumpectomy. So when I look at my chest it is a serious reminder of breast cancer. However, just the other day, I felt that this is not so bad after all. I think of the alternative, but mostly I think of all the women who have had such devastatingly awful diagnoses and treatments. I can't bitch about anything. So looking into the mirror I see the same old me, just more of me than I'd like. I need to shed some weight more than I need anything else. The illness is the problem to be dealt with, not the loss of a breast, or old age setting in (I'm 65).

jjensen

I think this is really about character, growth, strength, fears—the inner person we've become, and I still don't have an answer for it. My diagnosis was a wake-up call and I knew it. So who do I see in the mirror? A woman who is a work in progress: wiser than she was yesterday and not as wise as she will be tomorrow. But isn't that what life is all about, with or without breast cancer?

Mawsquaw

When I look in the mirror I see my mother looking over my shoulder giving me the strength and courage to continue the battle of everyday living and not to worry about the little things in life that I have no control over. Even though my mother has been gone for eight years to leukemia I feel she has been with me every step of the way. About a year after my diagnosis I had a dream in which I was told my cancer was back, so I went and talked to my mother about my diagnosis and in my dream she told me not to worry, that everything would be fine. Since that night I know I will be fine because my mother told me so.

pinkribbonsurvivor99

When I look in the mirror I see a patchwork girl. Someone who has fought hard for her life and has the scars to prove it. I see myself getting older and welcoming the changes. I look better than I have in a while as I am finally getting rid of the last chemo and tamoxifen weight. I see someone who will grow old and see my children grow up!

pinkwings

Pinkwings was first diagnosed when she was thirty-three and had a recurrence two years later; she is now in her forties. She and her husband adopted two little girls.

When I look into the mirror, I don't see the person I was before 1999. Before I retired in 1993 I was a very competent, independent, energetic, and tireless worker, and a helpful friend and neighbor. As an executive secretary I looked very polished in my appearance. Now, as I really look into the mirror, I see a person who has hair again but not as thick or pretty as it once was. This goes for my eyebrows and eyelashes as well. I look just a tad down from dumpy in my clothes. My beautiful shoe wardrobe is down to an old pair of sneakers and one pair of sandals. I realize these outward appearances don't really matter but they do affect one's self-image.

I have become more withdrawn from life due to the physical ailments and have become content to just hobble around the house. I do get out of the house to go to the various doctor visits, grocery shopping, and some errands. I have begun to use a cane, which helps. I don't mean this to sound so pitiful and debated writing it, but I wanted to be very honest. Think of it as a snapshot for today.

I do have so many things to be thankful for: God's grace and my coming through some difficult times, my husband's love, help, and support, and that of my family and friends. They are all so dear to me. Some of the decline in strength and health could be just part of aging. In closing, I want to say (I think it was Will Rogers who said it first) I have been through some terrible times in my life, some of which actually happened.

joy

I feel lucky that I can get up every morning and look in the mirror.

Jackjoy

When I look in the mirror I see a lady with more confidence and more fear. The confidence that comes from coping with troubles I never imagined would enter my life. The fear that comes from learning how hard it is for scientists to unlock the cancer riddle. I see a lady who never wanted to be associated with a "cause," and is still uncomfortable with the idea. I see someone who is enjoying life and appreciates the bonding to new friends who have come into her life because of breast cancer. I see someone who believes she has found the right balance between educating and taking care of herself and being proactive for the "cause," and yet not letting it take over her life.

Noel

I see myself, who I really am, for the first time. The illusion of who my parents/husband/daughter/friends/society expected me to be is gone. My body is more fragile than I ever knew, but my soul is stronger and more unwavering. There is a freedom in no longer trying to be perfect. I care less about what others think of me, and more about the mark I want to leave on this world.

happytobehere

When I look in the mirror I see myself as someone who has been fighting a *war* against a terrorist group called secondary breast cancer.

Small cell groups pop up in unguarded terrain and I have to start the fight all over again. I am very battle-weary with lots and lots of wounds, some deeper than others, but they all will heal and some will leave permanent scars. There won't be any medals or parades for me no matter how hard I fight but I will have the love of my family and friends as my reward. This is one fight I am going to win. *I will be the hero here, no matter what the outcome!*

When the media or people say "she lost the battle with cancer," they are using the wrong phrase. We don't ever lose the battle: we are the heroes in a war that we were never asked to be in but got dragged into kicking and screaming.

Cuddles

Cuddles was thirty-three when diagnosed with advanced breast cancer.

Whenever I bother to look in the mirror, which is not very often (my husband is always cleaning something off my face, like oil paint), I see an older me, 40 pounds overweight, gray hair, wrinkles . . . but I hardly ever see my scar. I don't know why, but it is probably because I've gotten so used to it I just don't notice it.

I don't like getting stared at by strangers, although at 65 I tend to be one of the "invisible ones" out there in the world. Unless I smile. Everyone reacts beautifully to smiles.

What I also see, is I still have laughter in my eyes. Fun kind of laughter, not ironic stuff. And hope, optimism, compassion for others, loyalty to my friends and family, and honesty. So I like what I see. Hey, it's me—I'm still here and not planning to be anywhere else very soon.

Annie Mac

Annie Mac, an artist, was first diagnosed in 1995 and died in 2006.

At the start of the cancer journey, the mirror was my enemy, pointing out defects, and after my mastectomy, I practiced daily looking in the mirror. At this time I was a sober woman, contemplating what was askew or deadly in me. I practiced smiling; in the past I was known to always have a smile on my face. I was one of those people who complete strangers will address out of a crowd, but the smile disappeared for a time. After a while, the smile was genuine again, and like Annie Mac, I stopped noticing scars. I stopped noticing tattoos. The scars are just a piece of me. The cancer is just a piece of me. Do I like it? No. I'd rather not have cancer, but I no longer see it as defining me and cancer did not rob me of my essence: I still am generally cheerful, I haven't lost a tendency to be a hothead, and I enjoy my same hobbies.

When I look in the mirror now, I generally see my smile and happy eyes. At times the sober me creeps in and when that happens I stand in front of the mirror for a very long time looking, searching deeply for what has slipped away. With the aid of the mirror, I find my self and gently draw her out.

Toni

In the past I was pretty shy and had anxiety issues over things like driving over a bridge. Now I see a woman who can get through anything. If I could get through two different types of breast cancer and their treatments, nothing will ever hold me back again. I see a woman who now thinks about the future. I see a smiling face and a healed soul who thanks God every day for watching over me.

flower girl

I am not sure what I see when I look in the mirror. Beyond the physical now that my boobs are gone and the reconstructive ones are there, I often wonder am I really still the same old me. No, I don't see that anymore. I do see a me that works harder now than ever to make it through each day and attempt to stay healthy. I see a me that wants to be happy and is now trying to find new ways to do so. I see a me that is still trying too hard to please others, job, daughter, family, etc. I see a me that needs to "re-find me."

Bonbon

I'm a person in progress and I was before breast cancer. But I think I just looked and didn't "see." The me I see today is physically different in several ways. I think I have to take my body as a whole. I have never defined myself by my breasts. The body loses and gains weight; I used to be tall (I lost almost 2 inches in height from all this); I'm gray-haired now (can't color it since I became allergic to hair color); and just recently gained a new biopsy scar on my right breast. The left breast is somewhat smaller because of the lumpectomy with a scar.

Emotionally it took some getting used to! We humans don't appreciate change much. So *who* I see emotionally is dramatically different than the *me* before breast cancer. I am sooo much wiser. I have learned I will never stop learning that being alive hurts and that is okay. I am much more relaxed and smile more. When I look in the mirror I *really* see me now—all of me!

Msnegs

I had a mastectomy 12 years ago, and was not a candidate for reconstruction. Even today, when I look in the mirror, it bothers me a great deal. I have gone beyond most of the negative thoughts of cancer, but when I go shopping for a new dress I get a little depressed because it is very difficult to find something that does not show up the scar and/or the mastectomy bra. Truly I feel lucky to be alive and am thankful for that, but a mastectomy does make it difficult to forget.

Rose Marie

Rose Marie was forty-nine when diagnosed.

I see myself. The same person I always was, only better. I'm one of those who say that breast cancer is the best thing to happen to me because of all the wonderful opportunities that have come to me and I've enjoyed. One year after diagnosis, surgery, chemo, radiation, and reconstruction, I became a Reach to Recovery volunteer. I tell anyone who asks, "If you've got a minute I can talk for an hour" about breast cancer. I'm livin' life and lovin' it.

asp

Asp was thirty-four when diagnosed.

Clothed or nude? I'm a reality-based woman. I see me, now with the scars and mutilation of breast cancer treatment. That's it.

Susana

In 1989 Susana had a double mastectomy.

I actually rarely look in the mirror to look at me. When I do look at me it's from the inside and that's the part I feel good about. That's the part that God sees. I've gotten way past what others think of me. I've long since realized I don't have to live up to their standards or expectations; believe it or not, for the most part we inject many of those standards and expectations on ourselves.

zoochild

When I look in the mirror I see a woman who has been changed by breast cancer (inside and out) and who will continue to change as long as she is alive. I have one breast and never had reconstruction done so I'll always look different than what's considered normal. It's been 17 years since my mastectomy, I've gone through losing and regrowing my hair 4 times with the recurrences (it's now grown back about 1 inch; I love it for the summer), I have a port-a-cath, and now during my last recurrence my spine has rounded and I no longer stand so straight with a nice flat back. So I see someone whose body shows the journey that she's been on. I believe that it has helped me and my family to be more compassionate toward others who may look different and deal with physical difficulties.

PCteacher

PCteacher was only thirty-two when diagnosed.

I see a woman of 47 looking as vibrant as when she was forty (of course I'm standing looking so the joint pain is at a standstill). I've always been "sick"; I've always been hospitalized. I had to deal with my mother dying during my recovery and I still survived. Every time I look at my flat tummy and my perky breast, I laugh at breast cancer: I got a free tummy tuck, breast lift, and I'm alive.

Lady Dee

CHAPTER FOURTEEN

Faith, Religion, and Spirituality

"People often say there are no atheists in foxholes; I suspect there aren't many in cancer wards, either."

2peke

None of the women here try to uncover the meanings of faith or godliness or proselytize; instead they write about their very personal connections to religion vis-à-vis their wish to have their breast cancer healed. Do things happen for a reason? If you believe that, then cancer is part of the larger picture of life, a test of your faith and your trust in God. And what about being on prayer lists? Is it just a case of "more is better"? Not to the women who are on multiple prayer lists in their community and nationwide; they take prayer lists very seriously. In this chapter the testimonials abound—about seeing angels, finding solace in churches and temples, even about the faith that comes from having highly competent doctors.

My own experience is almost laughable by comparison to the heartfelt entries that follow. I had just turned thirty-five and was being treated with surgery and radiation, and though my doctors were optimistic about my prognosis, I figured a little more help could only *be a good thing. I recall being in the Union Square Café in New York with one of my best friends when I swore I saw Bernie Siegel, author of* Love, Medicine and Miracles, *at the counter. Okay, that was Good Sign #1. Then by chance someone (the bartender?) showed me a rabbit's foot on a key chain—Good Sign #2. At that point I was convinced that if anyone suggested I stand on one leg, face west, and clutch the rabbit's foot while doing a visualization mantra such as "I will be fine, I will be fine," then all would be well in the world. Was I right? What can I say? I'm still here. Such is the power of faith, regardless of where you find it.*

> "Breast cancer has helped to fortify my
> strength."
>
> scrapper

PRAYER LISTS

There are many figures of speech associated with multiples: strength in numbers and birds of a feather readily come to mind. Accordingly, prayer lists offer tremendous hope for the woman who believes that the more prayer lists she's on the greater the possibility for healing.

After my second diagnosis, I was enrolled in 5 prayer groups across the country. Was I cured because of prayer? It couldn't hurt.
tuppie

> "Fear is an emotion, faith is a choice."
>
> Mawsquaw

When I was diagnosed, the way I told many people was to say something like "I need your prayers over the next months as I've been diagnosed with breast cancer." The night before my surgery, my dear husband and I were laughing about all the faiths I had praying for me: Catholics, Protestants, Jews, Muslims, Mormons, and Buddhists! My Internet buddies put me on prayer chains all over the country and even set up a prayer time at the time of my scheduled surgery so they would all be praying at the same time.

Little Dutch Girl

THINGS HAPPEN FOR A REASON

I never questioned "why me?" because I know that everything happens for a reason. I try to look at everything as an opportunity for spiritual growth, knowing that it is up to me and how I choose to handle adversity that makes the difference between calm acceptance and blind suffering. Breast cancer has helped to fortify my strength.

scrapper

I had friends tell me how amazed they were at my strength and how calm I was. I told them that I knew that God had a plan for me and that whatever the plan was, it was right for me. Twice over the past four years I have had an experience where I was very, very afraid. And suddenly a wave of calm just came over me. And in my head I heard words to the effect of "Why are you afraid? Trust in me." And that was it! I was once again calm.

junebug

I truly believe that there is a reason everything happens; we may not see it at first, but eventually we understand why. I am probably more religious now than I was before cancer and if someone were to say to me, there is no God, I would argue the fact. How can we look around us and how can we not believe in a higher being given the fact we are still here and living? Having cancer has made me smell the roses.

Marybe

SOMEONE TO WATCH OVER ME

Breast cancer made me aware of just how deep my faith is, and I discovered that I do absolutely trust God. No, that doesn't mean I won't have a recurrence, or possibly die from breast cancer. But I know God will be beside me every step of the way, and He will give me the strength to deal with whatever happens.

    kathi1964

I really do believe if most of us would just stand still and quiet for just a few moments we would feel God's peace and know that He is with us always.

    river

> "If breast cancer doesn't get you talking to God, then what will?"
>
>   lily987654

There's a great quote from a religious book I read during my chemo time. The author says that people view God as a crutch. Her response was, no, He's not a crutch—He's a whole hospital!!

    canuck

> "I see God in strangers that smile at me in passing."
>
>   1Faith

I am what you could call a "cradle" Catholic, and I belong to a very active parish. There have been numerous occasions where I've seen the hand of God at work in my life, but it's usually in hindsight that

I "get it." I find that when I'm trying to control everything in a given situation, that's when chaos reigns. I'm here to tell you that "Let go and let God" is no empty cliché.

metsfan

I too am a "cradle" Catholic and Black. When I was diagnosed I never prayed for a cure. I simply asked the Father to help me go through this in His will. Let some good come of this. As always, God answers prayer. There are a disproportionate number of minority women who get this disease. God allowed me to share the gift of "hope" with other women at my cancer center. I cannot tell you how grateful I am that God saw fit to turn my lemons into lemonade. Ain't God good?

Delivered

Faith is my doctor

My spiritual solace has come from my breast cancer support group and from my wonderful, compassionate doctors. I especially see God's hand in the doctors I have. (Most doctors who look at my surgical site whisper "beautiful." I smile every time it happens. Only a doctor could look at the disfigurement of a mastectomy and call it beautiful.)

Mawsquaw

> "I have a great deal of faith. I believe for me it's
> what has gotten me through the past few years.
> I think that if it works for you, stay with it."
>
> jealta

When I got my diagnosis I spoke with God about it and He told me He would walk beside me throughout my treatment. He led me to doctors who were compassionate and grounded in faith. When I needed spiritual support during the endless nights of nausea and vomiting and not being able to sleep, He led me to programs on TV which spoke to my heart and gave me peace and comfort. I read my Bible daily and each day I was shown passages that were a blessing to me.

rainbow

ANGELS: A STAIRWAY TO HEAVEN

Seeing angels beats sci-fi thrillers by a long shot, and for women who've experienced angels as apparitions, the result is a powerful curative.

I remember waking up from a dream with "Stairway to Heaven" playing which I hoped was not a bad omen. At Christmas Mass, I felt like I was the only one in the church and that the angels were surrounding me. The light just shone down on me and I felt protected and cherished.

newday

I too have seen my guardian angel. She first appeared to me shortly after my diagnosis and told me her name and that she was there to help me find "the stairway to heaven." At first I thought this meant I was going to die, but after much thought, I think it meant she was here to guide me through this process spiritually. I have seen her two other times, but only very briefly. I believe these images come to us when we are at our most vulnerable. I am not religious, but I have certainly become much more spiritual!!

maumau66

God let me know that He was with me and taking care of me by giving me a vision of an angel in my bedroom one night while I was sleeping. I awoke to a vision of an angel reaching out and touching me on my side as the touch of healing. This happened about 2 weeks after my diagnosis and I had not had any surgeries or treatments as of yet.

Lee

One morning I was lying in bed at my boyfriend's apartment looking up at the ceiling (and probably feeling sorry for myself) and I saw Jesus look down on me with his arms opened up. There were also angels. All of this was in the cottage cheese ceiling of the apartment. It was such an unreal experience. Later that day, try as I might, I couldn't see the angels or Jesus again in the ceiling. When I relayed the story to my mom, she began crying and I didn't know why. Years later she told me that her friend's daughter (a young women in her 30s with a 2nd diagnosis of breast cancer) was getting out of the shower when an angel tapped her on the shoulder. She died days later.

pinkwings

MIRACLE ON 34TH STREET

In the really bad times, when I was hospitalized after the chemo and alone in the room, I used to leave the Catholic channel on all night so the nuns would be with me and watch over me and not let anything bad happen. I remember the Christmas my son was in second grade and I was in the hospital and my oncologist had said my white count was so low I'd be there over Christmas. Carolers went up and down the hospital hall, but I couldn't see them because my door was closed. I could remember doing the same thing as a Girl Scout when we went to the hospital and sang to all the old people. Except I wasn't old now and this wasn't supposed to be happening to me. I couldn't even have the poinsettia the hospital put in every room. But my priest came to visit and like Christ raised Lazarus, Father raised my blood count. The oncologist sent me home

Christmas Eve, vowing he'd never, ever seen a white count rebound like that.

2peke

WE ARE ALL ONE

This is less of a religious catch-all than it is a reflection of the many venues women have found to offer some form of spiritual guidance and relief.

What religion is right? Can you worship and respect and not offend anyone? All religions are the same at their core—the struggle of many people. The struggle itself is the winning spirit of us mortals.

Eve

> "Faith is all of our middle name."
>
> artistic person

I have explored many more satisfying avenues of personal spiritual growth but at the expense of organized religion. I think both can coexist simultaneously.

Anne M.

I am currently experiencing heaven on earth, which really works for me because I do not believe there is a "hell."

Picassa

> "We all have different ways of seeking sanity and community."
>
> bradleyteach

I've always had a strong faith, but the love and support of other church members served to remind me that even though I am single, I am not alone.

kathi1964

I plan on catching the helicopter or rowboat, or whatever God sends my way in order to save my physical life and give me more time here with my family.

ally

Before I found out I was very sick with cancer I had spent four years in the process of becoming an Interfaith minister honoring all sacred paths. In the process of studying all the different religions I found myself to be Christian with a special connection to Buddhism. I believe God Is.

Greatful2b

I am a traditional Roman Catholic. I firmly believe that religion and faith is personal and one has to respect others' beliefs or lack of them. Because we lived abroad, we have friends of all faiths, so I was sent Tibetan chants to help me sleep (they did), Chinese liver charm bracelets, amulets, health charms, etc. Prayers sent on my name to mosques, temples, etc. I welcome all that because of the meaning for the person that was sending or doing this for me. But do not ever tell a cancer patient that they need faith and religion to get well because if treatments do not work that person thinks they were not religious enough or deserved to get well and that is very harmful.

dreamer

When I feel spiritually connected, I'm more at peace and better able to deal with whatever comes my way, even breast cancer!

HopeNFaith

A lot of you, if not most, have become more religious since breast cancer. And I am jealous of that. I am more spiritual I guess than religious. My eyes have been opened up more toward things like music, animals, nature, candles, and reading. We just need to find whatever it is that brings us comfort and helps us to heal, whether it is God or spirituality.

reginabu

"It's a home run!"

In my quest for some minute measure of control, I bargained with God. To use a sports metaphor, my one-sided conversation went something like this:

"Okay, you've got the playbook and you know how the game will turn out. I'm just getting tired of blindly running the plays! I don't want people at my funeral saying, 'Well, she managed to scratch out a couple more years after diagnosis, lucky girl.' Could you just give me a hint that all of this isn't going to be for nothing?"

Two days later, one of my oncology nurses who registered me for a clinical trial for herceptin called to tell me that not only was I randomized to get the trial med, but that I got on the longest arm of the study. There was my answer.

metsfan

"I Am the Light"

This is the name of a poem that Annie Mac especially liked. Her note is all the more poignant because she died in 2006, a little over ten years from the date of her original diagnosis.

I am not particularly religious in that I don't hold with any one "organized" belief system. But I do believe there is a higher power, God, something after this existence. I am even willing to accept the possibility of reincarnation for the purpose of learning what we were created to learn, whatever that is. I can accept the concept of karma, too. I felt for a long time that breast cancer had been visited upon me so that I could repay some karmic debts I'd collected. The year that I was first diagnosed and had the mastectomy, 1995, was the year that we lost our home/boat in a hurricane in St. Thomas, USVI (where we were living while I went through chemo); after the hurricane, when I could finally get a phone call out to my dad, I learned from him that he had cancer and only about 3 months to live. My husband and I, having nowhere to live anyway, went to live with my father. He died about 4 months later, and I was very fortunate to be with him at the time. So, I figured my "debt" was repaid.

Eight years later, here I am again, only this time the little cancer buggers are elsewhere in my body. What lesson must I learn now, I asked myself? There are several options, not the least of which is to be more willing to share myself with others.

I am not so afraid of death as I am sad to leave those I love.

Annie Mac

THE CALL OF THE WILD

For centuries people have drawn inspiration and comfort from the natural world— birding has got to be one of the gentlest outdoor "sports" I know of, second only to my favorite activity: listening to the ocean.

I don't consider myself a religious person. I too believe in a higher source and possibly reincarnation. I don't feel like I need to go to a church to feel closer to my higher source. When I got done with my chemo I left Iowa for a week and rejuvenated my spirit by spending a week on Vancouver Island with my best friend. We rented a cabin on the beach. Listening to the waves crash in the night made me closer to my higher source then I had felt in a long time.

B-Positive

CHAPTER FIFTEEN

Gathering Rosebuds

"My climbing rose reaches with joy for the sun."

Lizzi

When all is said and done—when the surgery is behind you, treatments have been given and pills swallowed, when your hair has grown back and your energy has returned—the question is, "What now? What do I do with today, the beginning of the rest of my life?"

Many years ago, when I was home between my junior and senior years in college, I learned that James, a high school boyfriend of mine, had cancer. I was devastated. It had not even been a year since my paternal grandfather had died from lung cancer and I had worshipped him. This news about my old boyfriend floored me: I was immobilized by fear. Fear of another death, of loving someone and losing him, and fear of something I didn't even understand. That summer I spent many days with James, sometimes hanging out with him after a chemo session or driving him places when he was too nauseous to take the wheel, or just going on long walks. And that summer I also made one fatal mistake: I didn't grasp how important his sense of time was, his need for joy and unconditional love. At a certain point James made his *case clear: it was his time to gather his rosebuds, and if I wasn't going to be part of his life looking ahead to the future, then I should step aside. I did, reluctantly.*

It is now some three decades hence: James is well and happy, and I am doing my best to gather my rosebuds, to do what's best for me first—not second, not last, not never. I am gathering my rosebuds now. Carpe diem, seize the day, live in the moment, be here now. It all makes perfect sense. In gathering all of these women in this book, I am gathering my fullest, most beautiful bouquet of rosebuds.

> "I *love* getting older as I truly know what the alternative is."
>
> pinkwings

SIMPLE PLEASURES

Simple Pleasures was the name of a little bakery shop on the South Fork of Long Island that I adored going to, especially in the summer. The smell of fresh bread, good coffee, and that first hit of sugar in the morning are all such simple pleasures, which is just another way of describing something direct, sensual, and very much in the here and now. It's hard to be unhappy about life when you bite down on a warm chocolate-filled croissant.

> "I really do stop to smell the roses."
>
> Number 1

I find that the more I can focus on the positive things and relationships that are important to me, the better I do. I also have a new appreciation of the small pleasures, in part because I fear I will lose them. This spring I have practically lived in my garden, really noticing the bees buzzing, the toads and frogs, the baby rabbits, and how my climbing rose reaches with joy for the sun.

Lizzi

I like the idea of just doing things that make you happy. It doesn't have to be anything on a grand scale level. Just simple things. I sometimes like to pet my cat and listen to her purr, read a book, or just pull the window up and watch and listen to the rain.

Jean

I have become so much more emotional in a good way as it takes little to make me cry. When I hold my grandchildren who were born after my breast cancer I am so thankful and have trouble holding back tears. Emotional health I believe is letting go of your emotions and experiencing life to the fullest. This month is my 5-year mark and that is so significant to me. I realize that I could get sick quickly but in the meantime life is to be enjoyed, including all the emotions that come along with it.

west coast woman

I like to run and I love the feeling after exercise, so I always make time for that. I do enjoy it if friends want to join me but if I need time alone I am honest and say so (another life skill I am getting better at).

Heather59

> "Most of us can get beyond the immediacy of having cancer and keep on living."
>
> songbird

I made a conscious decision eleven years ago to leave behind the corporate world and have never looked back. I removed the watch from my wrist and vowed never to wear one again. Painting and photography are passions of mine so I returned to school, got a second degree in visual arts, and now have a studio in my home that I love! The things I would like to have more time to do are simple: be with friends and family, make new friends, and simply sit back and relish in what I have rather than think about what I do not have. If you want to make changes in your life: do it! If you fear limited time to do it in: do it anyway!!! What is time anyway? Just a term, not a state of being.

Hummingbird

> "I sometimes need to remind myself that the 'new' me has new and different priorities."
>
> butterfly2

Friendship is a big part of enjoying life and relaxing

Another way of having fun is just getting together with a friend and the one who is hosting at her house has the table all set with a few lit votive candles for aromatherapy, some little tea cups, and a teapot of herbal tea. We turn some relaxing music on and just sit and "be." After a while we'll get to talking about something pleasant and just watch the flowers in her back yard. The next week she'll come over to my house and we'll repeat. Sometimes we just meet at the grocery store and browse through the aisles chatting and picking up a few things. These little pleasantries can make all the difference in one's day. If you don't have a good friend to do these things with you, do them alone—you'd be surprised how good it can make you feel.

googie

My breast cancer support group is blessed to meet at a pool at a four-star hotel! I haven't been able to go while I'm working, but I have the summer off. We swim every Wednesday and then always go out to lunch. A couple of us also meet at Starbucks now and then. We don't do many special things as a group, but I sure love these women. I also spend a lot more time doing *nothing* on the weekends, lying around with a good book, sitting in my yard . . . *not* running errands.

Agent99

"TUESDAY BELONGS TO ME"

If (when!!) you could make more time for the things you love to do most, for yourself, that makes you happy and fulfilled, whether ephemeral or as part of your legacy, what would they be?? Assume no time, financial, or other constraints—dream a bit and share your most favorite things to do.

Mine are (in no particular order): singing, listening to music, reading, birding and other nature observation, hiking, visiting the country's special places, needlecrafts, beading (rank beginner here), seeing musicals and plays and hearing concerts, playing a really fun board or card game, writing poetry and short fiction, exploring museums and historic sites, and traveling (top goals: Alaska, Greece, Scandinavia, Italy, Cayman Islands, and the Galapagos Islands).

songbird

I take every Tuesday for myself. I get up early and have my first pot of coffee, then I take myself to the little café that is close and have breakfast. I sit in front of the TV for a while, then I get ready to have lunch with my Rotary Club; after that I go shopping, not for anything special. Most of the time I don't buy a thing, but it is time that I spend with myself. I come home, have a glass of wine, my husband cooks supper, I sit and surf the web, then the day is done. Everyone in my household knows that Tuesday belongs to me and it better be an emergency if they want something. Before breast cancer I never took time for me; there just never was any. Now I make time.

Jackjoy

Several of the ladies I have met through this experience are planning a picnic this summer and a one-night "retreat"! I like to take long, hot baths with candles and bubbles; I also like to knit, but with chemo brain that is sometimes a little harder than it used to be. Irony of irony: I taught a group of high school girls at our school to knit and we knit chemo caps for ladies and men with cancer. I arranged for an oncologist to come out and speak with the girls. The next year, 11/2003, I was diagnosed. They knit me a cap and surprised me on my birthday with it! It was very special.

ally

MOVING FORWARD

My surgeon Peter Pressman told me that his goal is to help women move on from having to think about breast cancer. His job, he explained, is to make it possible for women to get on with their lives.

When we first got diagnosed, most of us said we were so scared/panicked, etc., that we could not eat, sleep, take in information, focus on our work, or much of anything, but once we got a grip on those immediate emotions and came to the understanding that we were not going to die right then, and we had a plan for what to do to move forward through our cancer treatment, we were able to resume focusing outside ourselves more and get back to living a fuller life. Not that there aren't setbacks, waves of uncontrollable fears, etc., along the way, but most of the time, most of us can get beyond the immediacy of having cancer and keep on living.

songbird

We should talk about how breast cancer may have shifted our ability to re-prioritize things in our lives. For me, it was very clear to not sweat the small stuff so to speak. I think after losing my mother, getting diagnosed soon after that, and managing a child with special needs, it was very easy for me to figure out the things in life that really are important. This truly was a benefit of receiving a cancer diagnosis. It gave me the opportunity to look at things in my life and place a true value on them without letting other non-essential things get in the way. How about you?

Eileen

Things I Love to Do:

1. Meet interesting people and learn all about them
2. Travel, travel, travel
3. Laugh with people, at myself. Laugh till I cry!
4. Hold my husband and children very tight
5. Learn new things every day!
6. Listen to live music (Try the New Orleans Jazz festival for serious sensory overload.)
7. Drink French Bordeaux
8. Gardening: weeding, pruning, planting, transplanting, sunburned neck, and tall glasses of lemonade
9. Reading a good book in a very comfortable chair that you can wrap your legs around
10. Hiking (Utah is awesome!)
11. Entertaining with lots of fanfare! (party games, sing-alongs, live music, mind-teasers, superb food, or even pajama parties for the girlfriends!)
12. Talking with God
13. Walking out of my many checkups with a clean bill of health.

Stormy

One thing this topic makes me think of is: to live as honestly as I can. This gives me such joy, though it's not always easy. I love my friendships and treasure the women in my life with whom I can share so much of myself, laugh, fight, make up, and be myself. I have always loved honesty in others and have strived to be that way myself, but since diagnosis something has definitely opened up in me. I'm just not as afraid to say what I feel and think, and not as worried about being judged for those feelings and thoughts. At times I've even found myself thinking: What's the worst thing that can happen to me by being truthful about this? I've already had cancer!!

For me it's a way of being in the world that has been liberating and wonderful. I think it's also a part of getting older . . . being more comfortable with oneself.

oceanwalker

Again, I feel (and, okay, it's different for me, because I'm thirteen years out) that breast cancer was a real blessing for me. It sure made me look at life a lot differently. It taught me to value family and friends and to savor every single moment I have with my child. It also taught me a lot about mothering. The only thing that got me through was the thankfulness that if this had to happen to somebody, it happened to me and not to my child. And I think if anyone was more devastated than I was, it was my mother.

2peke

"DO IT NOW"

You won't find the word procrastination *in the dictionary of a woman who's had breast cancer. Instead, the letter* p *stands for priorities, passion, personal, parents and parenting, play, peace, prayer, and pleasure.*

I used to spend a lot of energy on keeping my house perfect. Doing the spring and fall cleaning thing was essential. Now I can let things go (sometimes I have to because of my energy level) and it does not bother me as much. My standards are much lower than they used to be and I do not sweat the small stuff. When my daughter calls to go shopping or to the mall, I drop everything and go.

> Lee

My priorities have changed immensely. I moved from Texas, where I had lived a little over twenty years, back to my hometown to be closer to my family. I gave up a wonderful job and a house that I loved in doing this, but my family is much more important to me than those things. A job and home can be anywhere.

> SacredHeart

Enjoying life is where it's at. I sometimes need to remind myself that the "new" me has new and different priorities.

> butterfly2

Priorities seem to rearrange themselves after one has breast cancer. I know that was true for me and in the last 10 years of survivorship, I have a "Do It Now" list that keeps getting used daily.

> Dee

I really do stop to smell the roses.

> Number 1

There are only 24 hours in everyone's day. We can't manage to get more, but we can manage how we use them.

> butterfly2

"LIVE, LOVE, AND LAUGH!"

Once or twice a year, my friends from high school get together for an all-nighter. We go to a hotel or to a friend's house. Kick the kids or husbands out and bring out the food and drinks. We eat and drink almost all night long. (I usually end up falling asleep first!) We watch movies, call our friend in Italy, and just have a good ole' time. One time we did facials, another time we played games all night. Then in the AM we go out for a big breakfast. Even if it's only one or two friends, we try and get together. My husband and I now are trying to do more things by ourselves since our boys are old enough to be left home alone. Usually we come home to a mess, but so what. *Live, Love, and Laugh!*

> Purplepassion

Oh, my!! Live, Love, Laugh! That is my mantra. I found that on a small embroidered pillow right before I started chemo and bought it. I took it to every session (along with a fleece throw for warmth). Since then, I have become quite a collector of anything that expresses that thought. It is my goal in life. However, *life* is a work in progress and I do *love* many people (my grandchildren are at the top of the heap right now), yet the hardest part is the *laugh*. Even though we made jokes about each step of the way during the cancer thing, I seem to have lost the necessary focus. Thank you all for helping me! My license plate says "Llvluvlf." Lots of people guess "Live, Love, Life." I always say it works both ways.

> cj

I'm on a mission to add *fun* to the rest of the life I have to live.

> Msnegs

AGE IS BLISS

Ask any woman with this disease what she most wants and it invariably boils down to one word: tomorrow. *We want all our tomorrows and we want them for as long as possible, thank you very much. Getting older, especially having a birthday, is one of life's best vitamins for any woman getting over breast cancer.*

> "I'm the happiest 40-year-old on the planet,
> and I'll take every wrinkle and every gray
> hair gladly!"
>
> happytobehere

I am 64. Before my diagnosis I would get depressed over getting so old. I would never tell anyone my age. Now, I thank God that I made it another year (another Christmas, another birthday, etc.) and that I am so healthy and very, very happy.

I guess I have always been a very positive person (thanks to my Dad), but I find that I am even more so now. I really do stop to smell the roses. I am thankful for so many things, small things, daily. I stay away from negative people or people that make me feel bad. I am more forgiving—actually I am sounding so good I will probably go *straight* to Heaven. (I hope that I won't be all by myself and that everyone else will be down below having a ball!)

Number 1

It suddenly occurred to me that I no longer have a picture in my mind about being old. It's gone. I don't think about retirement or care about putting money away for the future. I used to.

Meta

I don't worry about it as much, because none of us know if we'll be here (it is so cliché, and I hate it, but it is true).

I still plan for the future. There are things I want to see/do/buy. But I don't obsess that we aren't saving a certain amount every pay day, like I used to. I tell myself we have to be fiscally responsible because I *will* be here when I'm seventy. I have more of an image of me "old" than I ever had before. Now that I think about, I never used to see myself as growing older. Now I do. I just pray that I can stay active.

Helen

After my recurrence, I really lived day to day. Then I started to think a week ahead, then a month ahead. I would have loved to have quit my job and spend every moment possible with my daughter, but there's no way I could afford it. Saving for retirement seemed like a ridiculous proposition. I used that money for time off and nice vacations instead. My long-term wish was to make it to 40. I thought asking for any more than that would be too outrageous a request.

Now I just turned 40 a couple of months ago, and I realize I need completely new goals! For the first time in eight years, I don't see limitations to my future. I'm thinking about how I'd like to spend my 50s, my 60s and beyond. At the same time, I still don't ever want to take any of it for granted.

On my birthday, a lot of people asked if I was sad about turning 40. I said absolutely not. I'm the happiest 40-year-old on the planet, and I'll take every wrinkle and every gray hair gladly!

happytobehere

Here, here! I agree with you fully. I found a gray hair this past Mother's Day and I smiled up to the heavens and thanked God!

I had a huge party for my 40th birthday last year. I had been warning my husband and family about it for years. My party was a Celebrate Life Party and we celebrated with a catered party of . . . banana splits!! It was fantastic and people talked about the party for weeks afterwards. The party celebrated my 40th, the official adoption of my 2 girls, and 5 years cancer-free. I am now 41 and thinking about my big 50th birthday party. I *love* getting older as I truly know what the alternative is. Here's to 50!!

pinkwings

I am so happy to be getting older, especially now. I am recovering from a liver metastasis. I am cancer-free again! At my 42nd birthday party this year one of my dear friends said "Thanks for being born."

Then my wonderful uncle said, "Better yet, thanks for staying alive!"
Here's to life!

    panthergirl

I don't think about getting older, just wiser.

    surviving soul

Afterword

This book is first and foremost a testament to the courage, openness, candor, and emotional generosity of the eight hundred women who participated in *First Person Plural*. It is also a testament to the perseverance and resolve of one woman, Ruth Peltason, who wanted to create the book she wished had been available at the time she most needed it. This book is also an example of technology living up to its promise, creating human connections online to call forth the very best in people.

Some of the women who participated in the *First Person Plural* online dialogue were veterans of excellent support groups and psychotherapy and had solid support networks of family and friends. Yet, whether they had other support structures or not, many of the women wrote that these dialogues allowed them to explore their joys and their challenges more profoundly, more thoroughly, and with more impact than anything they had done before.

None of the women whose voices are in this book would see herself as any more remarkable, insightful, or self-reflective than any other woman who has had to contend with breast cancer. Yet the *First Person Plural* dialogue allowed these women to join together in creating a uniquely powerful community, in which they very quickly found themselves inspired by one another to describe their most intimate experiences and share stories both painful and liberating.

How do eight hundred women engage in an intimate dialogue? And how do they do so on the Internet, a place not known for intimacy, for insight, or for powerful emotional experiences?

There were many things that contributed to the success of *First Person Plural,* but one essential element was the Small Group Dialogue technique that provided the structure for the online exchanges that are the heart of this book.

Small Group Dialogue (SGD) grew out of several decades of my experience using dialogues to create opportunities for people to wrestle with issues and ideas. As an independent filmmaker in the 1970s, I had had some wonderful experiences with audience discussions after film screenings. In the early '80s, I ran a not-for-profit organization called Media Network that specialized in training educators and activists to use films as discussion-starters in schools and community settings. After I created *P.O.V.,* a PBS series showcasing independent documentaries that were often provocative and controversial, I began looking for ways to encourage audience discussion of issues raised by *P.O.V.* films. In 1993, before there was a World Wide Web, we started to experiment with several basic techniques for online dialogues.

Most of the face-to-face discussions I'd been involved with in the 1970s and '80s came off well—some of them spectacularly well. The models for such discussions were fairly well developed. For example, we always began by asking people to introduce themselves. Just those short introductions shifted the dynamic immediately. Rather than some abstract representatives of various positions, you're encountering complex human beings who, like you, have been shaped by personal experiences. Even when the topic under discussion was highly emotional and people in the room disagreed, they made an effort to listen to one another.

But the first online dialogues we convened for *P.O.V.* had few of the elements of face-to-face discussions, and they were a mixed bag at best. Some—like a 1996 dialogue between people who had had profoundly different experiences during the Vietnam War era—were truly inspiring. I still remember the e-mail messages we received, from vets in particular, telling us how much they'd learned about themselves and about the people "on the other side," those who had opposed the war.

But other *P.O.V.* dialogues on controversial and emotional issues quickly deteriorated into what are often called "flame wars"—people talking at one another, insulting one another, even threatening one another. It was very unsettling, and clearly we had to come up with a better way.

In 1997, the Vietnam dialogue inspired me to transition out of *P.O.V.* to start Web Lab—a laboratory to expand the use of the Internet as a participatory medium—with the understanding that Web Lab would consult on *P.O.V.*'s online activities. After *P.O.V.*'s summer 1997 season (a season of too many flame wars), Web Lab took on the challenge of figuring out how to create high-quality discussions more consistently. By this point, the Web was well populated with chat rooms and other forums for discussion, but with few exceptions most online forums were at best a series of drive-by postings, and true dialogues, dialogues of any quality or depth, were all too rare. Barry Joseph, Web Lab's supervising producer, had a simple but brilliant idea: Why not adapt some elements of successful face-to-face discussions, combining them with the strengths of online discussions? Out of that idea the Small Group Dialogue technique was born.

The major features of SGD are:

Limited group size—Unlike large online forums, with hundreds or thousands of people posting at random but never really engaging one another, SGD assigns participants to small groups, each with a limited number of members. In the case of *First Person Plural*, for example, instead of eight hundred women posting in one space, we had twenty groups with forty members each.

Anonymity with accountability—Participants can create screen names to preserve the safety that anonymity provides, although they are asked to post short bios and introduce themselves when the dialogue kicks off. People get to know one another quickly.

Discussions unfold over time—Unlike chat rooms, where everyone must be online at the same time, SGD is an "asynchronous" dialogue, sometimes called a bulletin board. Posts are organized by topic and available for reading at any time. Members can write responses whenever they log on, day or night, and take whatever time they need to compose their messages. Conveners can suggest topics, but also encourage participants to create whatever topics are of interest to them. Participants have the option to post in as few or as many topics as they want.

Limited duration—Participants are told at the outset that the dialogue will have a limited initial time frame, in this case two weeks. Members of each group start together and come to closure together. Limiting the duration encourages higher levels of participation and a more intense group experience.

Over the course of several years, with discussions about controversial, often emotional topics, such as the Clinton impeachment, race, and the impact and implications of September 11, the results were extraordinary. Not only did SGD eliminate flame wars, many participants found that their participation was a transformative experience.

In 1997, several people had suggested that the Vietnam dialogue would make a very powerful book. The timing wasn't right then, but by 2002, after several years of successful Small Group Dialogues, I wanted to create a series of online discussions that could be edited into a unique set of books. Given her many years as a book editor, I asked my friend Ruth Peltason what she thought of the idea. She was immediately enthusiastic and we began to brainstorm possible topics. A few days later, she said, what about making the first one about breast cancer?

Until then, SGD had been used mostly for what we called "dialogues across differences"—respectful explorations of divisive political or cultural issues. Although sharing experiences about breast cancer is neither contentious nor controversial, it seemed like SGD would be a great fit just the same. The anonymity and the structured discussions, as well as the intimacy they foster, create such a feeling of community and safety.

As it turned out, *First Person Plural* went beyond anything we could have imagined. Like any life-threatening or life-changing experience, breast cancer calls up a range of powerful, confusing, sometimes overwhelming feelings: mortality, body image, what it means to be a woman. Many people would rather not "go there." By providing a powerful opportunity for women to find kinship and support, as well as a unique sense of safety and intimacy, Small Group Dialogue gave the women of *First Person Plural* an opportunity they had found nowhere else: to describe sometimes painful, sometimes terrifying experiences. In so doing, many women recalibrated their sense of themselves and discovered the full measure of their own strength and resilience. And, as the women themselves have said in so many ways, out of that process came insight, self-knowledge, and even an unexpected kind of joy.

It is an honor to be able to share their insights and inspiration with the much wider audience of women, their families, friends, and caregivers who will read this book.

Marc N. Weiss

List of Breast Cancer Organizations

We thank the following organizations for their support in this project.

breastcancer.org is a nonprofit organization dedicated to providing the most reliable, up-to-date, and complete breast cancer information for women and their loved ones. The website offers physician-reviewed information on breast cancer research, prevention, detection, treatment, and recovery; monthly educational programs; updates on research breakthroughs; and is where people affected by breast cancer can connect with each other.

breastcancer.org | 111 Forrest Avenue, 1R | Narberth, PA 19072 | Phone: 610.664.1990 | www.breastcancer.org

Breast Cancer Action carries the voices of people affected by breast cancer to inspire and compel the changes necessary to end the epidemic.

Breast Cancer Action | 55 New Montgomery, Suite 323 | San Francisco, CA 94105 | Toll-free number: 1.877.2STOPBC | www.bcaction.org

The Breast Cancer Research Foundation® is dedicated to preventing breast cancer and finding a cure in our lifetime by funding clinical and genetic research worldwide. A minimum of 85 cents of each dollar donated to the foundation goes directly to breast cancer research and awareness programs.

The Breast Cancer Research Fund | 60 East 56th Street, 8th floor | New York, NY 10022 | Toll-free number: 866.FIND.A.CURE | www.bcrfcure.org

FORCE: Facing Our Risk of Cancer Empowered is the only national nonprofit organization devoted to improving the lives of individuals and families affected by hereditary breast and ovarian cancer. FORCE provides information, support, awareness, advocacy, and broadcast updates on hereditary breast and ovarian cancer research.

Facing Our Risk of Cancer Empowered | 16057 Tampa Palms Blvd. W, PMB #373 | Tampa, FL 33647 | Toll-free number: 888.288.7475 | www.facingourrisk.org

The **Intercultural Cancer Council** (ICC) promotes policies, programs, partnerships, and research to eliminate the unequal burden of cancer among racial and ethnic minorities and medically underserved populations in the United States and its associated territories.

Intercultural Cancer Council | 1709 Dryden, Suite 1025 | Houston, TX 77030-3411 | Phone: 713.798.4617 | www.iccnetwork.org

Living Beyond Breast Cancer is a national nonprofit education and support organization dedicated to empowering all women affected by breast cancer to live as long as possible with the best quality of life. Programs and services include interactive conferences; teleconferences; an informational website; quarterly newsletters; publications for medically underserved women; low-cost informational recordings; networking programs; workshops and trainings for health-care providers; and the Paula A. Seidman Library and Resource Center.

Living Beyond Breast Cancer | 10 East Athens Avenue, Suite 204 | Ardmore, PA 19003 | Survivors toll-free help line: 1.888.753-LBBC | www.lbbc.org

The Mautner Project improves the health of lesbians, bisexual, and transgender women who partner with women and with their families through advocacy, education, research, and direct service.

The Mautner Project | 1707 L Street, N.W., Suite 230 | Washington, D.C. 20036 | Toll-free number: 866.MAUTNER | www.mautnerproject.org

Sisters Network® Inc. (SNI) is the only national African-American breast cancer survivorship organization in the U.S. SNI promotes the importance of breast health through empowerment, support, breast education programs, resources, information, and research.

Sisters Network Inc. | National Headquarters | 8787 Woodway Drive, Suite 4206 | Houston, TX 77063 | Toll-free number: 866.781.1808 | www.sistersnetworkinc.org

Y-ME National Breast Cancer Organization's mission is to ensure, through information, empowerment, and peer support, that no one faces breast cancer alone. Y-ME has the only 24-hour hotline staffed entirely by trained breast cancer survivors, with interpreters in 150 languages. Affiliates provide services such as support groups, early detection workshops, wigs and prostheses for women with limited resources, and advocacy on breast cancer-related policies in their communities.

Y-ME National Breast Cancer Hotline | 800.221.2141 (English) | 800.986.505 (Spanish) | www.y-me.org

The Young Survival Coalition (YSC) is the premier international, nonprofit network of breast cancer survivors and supporters dedicated to the concerns and issues that are unique to young women with breast cancer. Through action, advocacy, and awareness, the YSC seeks to educate the medical, research, breast cancer, and legislative communities, and to persuade them to address breast cancer in women 40 and under. The YSC is a point of contact for young women living with breast cancer.

Young Survival Coalition | 61 Broadway, Suite 2235 | New York, NY 10006 | Toll-free number: 877.YSC.1011 | www.youngsurvival.org

Acknowledgments

This book is the result of two journeys, each of them long in the making: first, it is the collective voice of hundreds of women, and second, it is inspired by my own personal experiences with breast cancer.

My deepest thanks go to the women who are the heart and soul of this book. I wish that I could give each one a hug of thanks. They changed my life. I now have eight hundred new friends who come from all over the world, and they are as fine a group of women as one might ever meet. Over the course of this project, some of the women died from their illness; how ironic and sad that each was someone whose comments burst with personality and goodness. I will never forget them.

When I had the idea for this project, I felt that Marc Weiss would be a strong and caring partner, and indeed he was. Marc is not one to do things halfway, and his commitment was palpable; it was his mojo that was instrumental in getting part one of this book project—the actual Web program called *First Person Plural* (FPP)—off the ground. Our fairy godmother in this venture was Amy Langer, former director of NABCO among her scores of credentials. Amy was referred to us by Peter I. Pressman, and she was both adviser and worker bee. We learned so much from her.

The learning curve is steep for a project as complex as this, and to help guide us we partnered with ten leading breast cancer organizations, each of whom was an active adviser and also offered links to our Web project on their websites. These organizations—and indeed others like them—carry on the emotionally difficult but necessary work of helping women everywhere deal with breast cancer disease. For our project I commend and deeply thank breastcancer.org, Breast Cancer Action, FORCE, the Intercultural Cancer Council, Living Beyond Breast Cancer, the Mautner Project: The National Lesbian Health Organization, NABCO, Sisters Network, Y-ME National Breast Cancer Organization, and Young Survival Coalition. In particular I wish to single out Janine Guglielmino, Elyse Caplan, and Jean Sachs at LBBC and Lara Marek at breastcancer.org for their gracious help and time.

To the Web Lab staff, I offer my sincere thanks. On the subject of staff, I need to single out Elaine Hunt, whom I first met online when she served as dialogue manager of the FPP website. A couple of years later when I was knee-deep in piles of posts and comments to wade through and edit for the book, Elaine responded to my e-mail query for help. Elaine lives in Canada, I am in New York, and yet I felt we were connected at the hip; though she pretended to be my assistant, in truth, Elaine was a true partner and adviser. As I often said to her, I would not have been able to do this book without her.

In developing the website, my thanks to Judy Richland of Richland Design Associates, who not only designed our website but made it look so happy and fresh and gave it such a nice raspberry color. The "face" of *First Person Plural* was aptly and adorably conveyed in illustrations by the equally adorable and lovable Maira Kalman. Maira typically does not allow her art to "illustrate" any work other than her own, so we were indeed fortunate when she allowed us to reproduce some images for the website. My gratitude is stratospheric.

In realizing this book, I had two earthly angels at my side: my agent, Alice F. Martell, and my lawyer, Jaime Wolf. Alice's confidence in me and enthusiasm for this book has given me buoyancy beyond measure—equal, in truth, to my gratitude to her. Alice is an author's best friend, and she absolutely made this book happen. Let me repeat this for emphasis: Alice made it happen. Kudos also go to my friend Jaime Wolf, the most darling of diplomats. Not only does Jaime have the keenest of legal minds, he dispenses lawyerly advice with balletic grace. His help was peerless and touching.

Alice sent my proposal to Henry Ferris, executive editor at William Morrow, who she holds in high esteem. I can see why. Henry is gifted. Not only did he come up with the best title for this book (truly a blind spot of mine), but his suggestions for the text were always spot-on, and where I couldn't see what was needed, Henry did, with an editor's 20/20 vision. For his je ne sais quoi touch, I am immensely grateful. Aja Pollock is this author's blessed copy editor: Aja's quiet strength is a combination of careful reading and a deft touch.

Although this book isn't about me, my position as its emcee is a result of my personal encounter with breast cancer. Those who know me will not be surprised that I begin these thanks with my doctors, each of whom I hold in high esteem. There is my internist, Mitchell Adler, who suggested when I was thirty-five that I see Julie Mitnick, M.D., for a mammogram; looking back I would be pressed to find more prescient counsel. Julie and I formed a bond at that first appointment, and to say I trust Julie with my life is no overstatement. Julie's diminutive height of barely five feet belies her greatness in the field of radiology, for she is a towering figure of skill and compassion, something she excels in day after day, with thousands of women, over the years. I have been blessed with her beaming smile that signals the "all okay" reading, and I have been touched by the grace and compassion with which she has given me troubling news from time to time. There is the irrepressible, irresistible, and immensely gifted surgeon Peter I. Pressman, M.D., whom Julie recommended. Indeed, the word *surgeon* is inadequate for citing his many achievements. When we met in 1990 I was taken in by Peter's brilliance, innate self-confidence, and bonny personality. Why are surgeons derided for lacking a bedside manner? I'll never be able to answer that one, for each time following a surgery it was Peter who came to see me in the hospital, offer comfort, explain a diagnosis. I'm a fairly proactive patient, and never once did he shy away from a spirited discussion or make me feel he was too busy for me. I am proud (though still a bit uncomfortable!) that he now asks me to address him by his first name. For keeping me well and well informed, and for so much more, I thank him from the bottom of my heart. I am honored that he agreed to write the foreword to this book. And where there is Peter, there is also Peggy, his wife and former office manager. Peggy is a dear soul with natural warmth who always gave me such hope when I came for appointments. For sheer behind-the-scenes calm and care, I thank Bruce Deitchman, M.D. What began as a doctor-patient relationship (he was my dermatologist) has turned into a special friendship. Bruce's former work as a pathologist specializing in breast cancer meant that he was able to help me puzzle out pathology reports and focus on the important issues. To this day, he deflects my worry with humor and intelligence. His encouragement in my endeavor to do this book has been enormous and constant. For rebuilding that platform formerly known as my chest, I owe my décolletage to Gregory LaTrenta, M.D., an artist at reconstruction and a truly nice man. As every woman with breast cancer knows, after a point the starring role in one's care goes to the oncologist, and in this regard I am indeed fortunate to be treated by the great Anne Moore, M.D. When she listens—which she does like no one else—Dr. Moore sort of leans forward, her intent face and body language reinforcing the interest she shows in a patient; I am continually awed by her brilliance. She, too, encouraged my efforts in making this book and led me to believe it was a worthy undertaking. In Dr. Moore's office I want to thank the two Pats: Patricia Farrell, the knowing and always kind oncology nurse, and Pat Tortorici, who used to manage the blizzard of calls and schedules for Dr. Moore. Also overseeing my care has been Caryn E. Selick, M.D., my ever-vigilant gynecologist and friend since my mid-thirties, as well as her wonderful nurse assistant, Rebecca Emel. Alan Hack, Ph.D., who guided me through shoals imaginary and otherwise, continues to make it possible for this patient to feel healthy inside and out.

I am blessed to have so many friends, and there are two women in particular who have made the entire journey with me—Nancy Meyer and Amy Lesser Courage. We all grew up in St. Louis, and whether that fueled their devotion in the to-and-fro of my illness, I can't say. But I do know that they are my sisters and I love them deeply. They mean the world to me. Nancy, who has uncommon wisdom and compassion, is the most generous human being I have ever been privileged to know. As she likes to say, hers is an "old soul," and bless her for that—may we continue to age and grow old together. Nancy's encouragement in regard to this project can neither be measured nor overstated, and I can't thank her enough. As for Amy—! Her sparkling optimism, loyalty, and unstinting friendship have been a balm again and again. How many times have I awakened to her welcoming presence in the recovery room, or heard her cheery voice on the phone after a procedure? How many times has she simply "been there"? Lucky, lucky me.

There are so many others to whom I owe a thousand bows. I thank Laura Jacobs and Jim Wolcott (their keen reading of parts of my text was especially helpful), Ana Rogers and Gene Seidman, Robert and Bezo Morton, Susan Murcko, Emily Benton Morgan, Kate Jamison, Donna Torrance, Todd Dimston, Charlene Bry, Danny Meyer, Nori Obata, Julia Leach, Susan Anthony, Lavinia Grimshaw, Gabriella De Ferrari, John Taylor and Dianne Dubler, Daphne Lingon, Susan Hager and Adrian Alganaraz, Judy Hudson, Page Goolrick, Brenda Cullerton, Daniel Aronstein, Judith Michael, Rifka Schoenfeld, John Russell, and my cousins, Lynn Newman and Paul Steinbaum . . . it's a long list of many wonderful people. I trust they each know their unique gifts to me. A special mention of my love and gratitude goes to Paul Gottlieb, former president of Harry N. Abrams, Inc., Publishers, where I worked for many years. Paul showed me unusual empathy and understanding when I was dealing with breast cancer, and no employee could have had a more sympathetic boss. He also introduced me to Evelyn Lauder, who took me under her capable wing and helped me in my quest to learn more about this disease and get well. Not only did Evelyn in time become an author, but she became a friend, and I am privileged to know her. I am also indebted to Evelyn for her belief in this project, and I applaud her many times over.

The ease in writing my thanks comes to a full stop when I must acknowledge my parents and two brothers and sister-in-law. How does one thank in public what is the naturally private world that family inhabit? From my father, who died before my recurrence, I received calming support (he also tried to convince me to move back to St. Louis, but that's another story). My mother has always shown me steadfast care and concern, and shed more than her fair share of tears along the way. It is often said of parents that they would take a bullet for their child. I don't know that my mother would have swapped places with me in the O.R., but she certainly wished she could have mitigated my pain many times along the way. Her love and support are very important to me. In their inimitable ways, my older brothers were both special. Jim had an amazing ability to remember each doctor visit, and his calls to check on me afterward were reassuring, even though I endured a fair amount of teasing along the way. As for Charlie, the oldest, he has been my big brother and best friend every single step of the way over these long years. In another life Charlie must have been a caregiver. To see his smiling face and feel the warm pressure of his hand in mine after a surgery remains one of my most tender memories. Although I have only one sister-in-law, I'm fond of saying that Barbara Peltason is my *favorite* sister-in-law. And it's true. She is 100 percent wonderful. Above all, I treasure the week she came to New York to help me after a surgery. There were moments both comical and dark, and I hope that like me she only remembers the good bits.

Over the years there has been one woman, a friend and former colleague of mine, who has been in my back pocket, so to speak. Elissa Ichiyasu and I met when we were both starting out—I was an editorial assistant at Knopf and Elissa was a rookie designer at Pantheon, a sister company. We worked together on a project or two.

Many years later we were both at Abrams, each further along in our careers and life. Again, we worked together on books. One day I commented that her hair looked different and she confided in me that it was a wig. She had breast cancer. Six months later so did I. We also had the same doctors. But here the similarities end, for when Elissa had a recurrence it was fatal. I like to imagine that she would like this book; I like to imagine how she would have designed it, for she was the deftest of book designers. I began missing Elissa even before she died, and I miss her still. In part, this book is a tribute to Elissa and her bravery.

Of heavenly angels, I have three: my darling grandmother, Ruth M. Peltason; my aunt, Ellen Peltason Steinbaum Wallerstein; and the woman who was like a second mother to me, Willie Mae Gray. Although only my aunt was alive in the years dating from my first diagnosis, each, in her own way, has been an inspiration and a comfort to me, and each offered me that rarest of gifts: unconditional love.